AGEING IN SUB-SAHARAN AFRICA
Spaces and practices of care

Edited by

Jaco Hoffman and Katrien Pype

D1612577

First published in Great Britain in 2018 by

Policy Press
University of Bristol
1-9 Old Park Hill
Bristol
BS2 8BB
UK
+44 (0)117 954 5940
pp-info@bristol.ac.uk
www.policypress.co.uk

North America office:
Policy Press
c/o The University of Chicago Press
1427 East 60th Street
Chicago, IL 60637, USA
t: +1 773 702 7700
f: +1 773 702 9756
sales@press.uchicago.edu
www.press.uchicago.edu

British Library Cataloguing in Publication Data
A catalogue record for this book is available from the British Library

Library of Congress Cataloging-in-Publication Data
A catalog record for this book has been requested

ISBN 978-1-4473-2526-0 paperback
ISBN 978-1-4473-2525-3 hardcover
ISBN 978-1-4473-2528-4 ePub
ISBN 978-1-4473-2529-1 Mobi

Cover design by Policy Press
Front cover image: Shutterstock
Printed and bound in Great Britain by CMP, Poole
Policy Press uses environmentally responsible print partners

To several pioneers of research on ageing in Sub-Saharan Africa:
Nana Araba Apt, Maria Cattell, Monica Ferreira,
Morag Insley, Valerie Møller and Sjaak van der Geest.

Contents

Lists of photos, figures and tables

Photos

Figures

Tables

Notes on contributors

Andries Baart, Professor emeritus, Ethics of Care and Chair, Presence and Care. Since 1991 he had full professorships at several universities in the Netherlands and currently is Extraordinary Professor, Optentia Research Focus Area, Vaal Triangle Campus, North-West University, South Africa. He is the father of the theory of presence and undertakes intensive field, theoretical and foundational research in the broad area of care, wellbeing and service provision. In this regard, his research particularly focuses on the socially vulnerable and the ethics of care.

Josien de Klerk, Lecturer (global public health), Leiden University College, The Hague. Josien has worked extensively on ageing in the era of AIDS in Kenya and Tanzania, looking at informal care, including self-care of both affected and infected older people in rural and urban settings. Her fieldwork is the basis of critical analysis of the politics around ageing and care in the treatment-dominated AIDS landscape in East Africa.

Emily Freeman, Assistant Professorial Research Fellow, London School of Economics (UK) and Political Science as well as Visiting Senior Research Fellow at the Optentia Research Focus Area, NorthWest University, Vaal Triangle Campus (South Africa). Emily's research focuses on ageing, care and sexual health in Sub-Saharan Africa. She has worked extensively on HIV in older age in Malawi and her current research considers new possibilities for formal care in older age across the region. A recent important publication is one with E Coast in 2014, Sex in older age in rural Malawi, which was published in *Ageing and Society*.

Jaco Hoffman, Associate Professor, Optentia Research Focus Area, North-West University, Vaal Triangle Campus (South Africa), and James Martin Senior Research Fellow, Oxford Institute of Population Ageing, University of Oxford (UK) where he coordinates the African Research on Ageing Network (AFRAN). He is also Honorary Research Fellow at The Albertina and Walter Sisulu Institute of Ageing in Africa, University of Cape Town, South Africa. Jaco's research particularly focuses on ageing through the life-course and intergenerational dynamics in the context of poverty and HIV/AIDS in South Africa. A related publication is an article with Isabella Aboderin in the *Canadian Journal of Aging* (2015) on 'Families, Intergenerational Bonds, and Aging in Sub-Saharan Africa'.

Brigit Obrist, Professor of Anthropology, University of Basel, Switzerland, and the Swiss Tropical and Public Health Institute. Brigit currently leads a medical anthropology research group in the fields of migration and urban health, sexual and reproductive health, ageing and health, media and health, addressing infectious, non-communicable as well as neglected diseases. A recent publication is, *Living the City in Africa*, which she edited with Veit Arlt and Elisio Macamo.

Katrien Pype, Assistant Professor, Institute for Anthropological Research in Africa, Katholieke Universiteit Leuven (Belgium), and Birmingham Fellow, Department of African Studies and Anthropology, University of Birmingham (UK). Katrien's main research interests are popular culture and technology and society interactions which led to a postdoctoral research project on how older people live in Kinshasa – a heavily mass-mediated urban environment. Several articles (in among others, *Ethnos: Journal of Anthropology*; and *Journal of African Cultural Studies*, both 2017) and book chapters (in *Everyday Media Culture in Africa: Audiences and Users*, co-edited by W. Willems and W. Mano, Routledge, 2016) are forthcoming.

Sjaak van der Geest, Professor Emeritus, University of Amsterdam, and visiting professor at BRAC University in Dhaka, Bangladesh and Gulu University, Uganda. Sjaak's fieldwork includes a wide variety of subjects, for example, sexual relationships and birth control, the use and distribution of medicines, popular song texts, meanings of growing old. He has written extensively, has been editor of numerous books and also founded the journal *Medische Antropologie* and was its editor-in-chief for more than 20 years.

Peter van Eeuwijk, Professor, Institute of Social Anthropology, University of Basel, Institute of Social Anthropology, University of Zurich (Switzerland), and the Swiss Tropical and Public Health Institute. Peter is a social anthropologist engaged as senior lecturer and senior researcher in medical anthropology, anthropology of ageing, urban anthropology, engaged anthropology, political ecology and sustainable development. Two important publications of his are: 'Pains, pills, and physicians: self-medication as social agency among older people in urban Sulawesi, Indonesia', which appeared in an edited volume *Alter(n) anders denken: Kulturelle und biologische Perspektiven* published in 2013 by Böhlau, and an article published in 2014, 'The elderly providing care for the elderly in Tanzania and Indonesia: making "elder to elder" care visible', in *Sociologus*.

Series preface

Series editors: Chris Phillipson (University of Manchester, UK),
Toni Calasanti (Virginia, Tech, USA) and
Thomas Scharf (University of Newcastle, UK)

As the global older population continues to expand, new issues and concerns arise for consideration by academics, policy makers and health and social care professionals worldwide. *Ageing in a Global Context* is a series of books, published by Policy Press in association with the British Society of Gerontology, which aims to influence and transform debates in what has become a fast-moving field in research and policy. The series seeks to achieve this in three main ways: first, through publishing books which re-think key questions shaping debates in the study of ageing. This has become especially important given the re-structuring of welfare states, alongside the complex nature of population change, both of these elements opening up the need to explore themes which go beyond traditional perspectives in social gerontology. Second, the series represents a response to the impact of globalisation and related processes, these contributing to the erosion of the national boundaries which originally framed the study of ageing. From this has come the emergence of issues explored in various contributions to the series, for example: the impact of transnational migration, cultural diversity, new types of inequality, and contrasting themes relating to ageing in rural and urban areas. Third, a key concern of the series is to explore inter-disciplinary connections in gerontology. Contributions will provide a critical assessment of the disciplinary boundaries and territories influencing the study of ageing, creating in the process new perspectives and approaches relevant to the 21st century.

Given the ambitions of the series, the editors are delighted that one of the early contributions focuses on issues relating to older people living in Sub-Saharan Africa (SSA). Jaco Hoffman and Katrien Pype have brought together an impressive group of contributors to explore issues of urgent concern to the development of health and social policy in SSA. The various chapters draw together ethnographic, survey and policy-related material, exploring different aspects of family-based care in SSA. The book represents a major achievement and will be essential reading for academics, NGOs, and policy makers more generally.

Acknowledgements

Ten years since the establishment of the African Research on Ageing Network (AFRAN) under the leadership of Isabella Aboderin and Jaco Hoffman at the Oxford Institute of Population Ageing, University of Oxford, the publication of this volume in the British Society of Gerontology 'Ageing in a Global Context' series is part-testimony that ageing research in Sub-Saharan Africa is coming of age. This coming-of-age story is about the transcendence from essentialist notions of Africanness to analysing the complexities of contemporary Africa where modernity and traditionalism do not constitute mutually exclusive categories; where the uncritical embrace of a linear modernisation and ageing theory as explanatory framework is critiqued by nuanced in-depth grounded analysis; where ageing research on the youngest continent is part of a new global discourse about what constitutes a 'good' and 'affordable' old age.

Generously funded by the Marie Curie IOF (PIOF-GA-2009-252331) and Newton Alumni Scheme, the contributors were in a position to extensively discuss their contributions at a colloquium convened by Katrien Pype at the University of Leuven. The editors and authors want to thank the participants, in particular Vera Roos, Nadia Fadil, Filip De Boeck, Thomas Hendriks, and Steven Van Wolputte for their valuable and detailed comments. In addition, the anonymous reviewers invited by the publishers also contributed with constructive suggestions on the volume in general and chapters in particular.

The editors and authors are furthermore grateful to Amanda Diener and Isabelle de Rezende for excellent editorial and administrative assistance, which is not taken for granted and much appreciated. This appreciation also goes for financial support − in addition to the funding agencies already mentioned − to North-West University (Optentia Research Focus Area), University of Antwerp (VLIR-UOS funding) and the Swiss National Science Foundation (SNSF).

Introduction:
Spaces and practices of care for older people in Sub-Saharan Africa

Jaco Hoffman and Katrien Pype

Background

Globally, life expectancy at birth has increased by more than 30 years over the last century (Roser, 2015). A major difference between population ageing in the more developed and the still developing regions of the world is that ageing in the latter largely takes place against a backdrop of considerable economic, infrastructural and personal strain, with the family seen as the main (if not the only) source of care. Longevity, even when achieved, often means a life of compromised health with scant access to general (let alone appropriate or specialised) care and similarly constrained financial resources. These additional years, which in the more developing parts of the world do not necessarily translate into healthy longevity, challenge individuals, families, civil society and the state in terms of the social and health care of its older members. However, though much has been achieved in terms of prevention and treatment, accompanying the longevity revolution is an added imperative: understanding and developing a culture of care that is sustainable, affordable, compassionate and universal is critical (Aboderin and Hoffman, 2012).

Despite remaining younger than all the other world regions, Sub-Saharan Africa (SSA) is seeing its older populations similarly growing in absolute numbers – its current population of 44 million aged 60 and over is expected to increase fourfold to 160 million in 2050 (UNPD, 2012). Although people age in a diverse range of settings across the continent, most care for older people in SSA is provided by families, typically in settings of entrenched poverty and infrastructural constraints. Yet, debate on the experience of caregiving *for* older people and its implications for policy in the region is virtually non-existent, and there is very little active discussion and exploration of what the relative care roles and responsibilities of families, the state and other sectors ought to be.

In contexts of poverty (youth unemployment) and HIV/AIDS in particular, concern (especially in southern Africa) has focused on the economic and social costs of care provided *by* older to younger generations (Barrientos et al, 2003; Madhavan, 2004; Ardington et al, 2010). Yet little attention has been paid to questions of care *for* older people. Who will care for the carers?

As part of an intensifying research endeavour on ageing and health in SSA, findings of a few representative surveys have actually highlighted a significant prevalence of functional impairment and disability – and a need for long-term care for SSA's older populations – while a handful of recent small-scale studies have begun to investigate its actual patterns and experiences (Cassim et al, 2012; Phaswana-Mafuya et al, 2012). Though limited, the available empirical evidence shows profound inadequacies in familial care provision; major economic, mental and physical caregiver strain; and a clearly emerging demand for 'formal' community care services.

These apparent realities of long-term care have, to date, received little if any consideration in current policy agendas addressing the issue. Instead, frameworks still underline the family as asset and promote the exclusive role of family care, thus reflecting a broader, largely uncontested, policy and public discourse on 'traditional' African family values as a bedrock for progress and 'homegrown' development on the continent. This overriding 'official discourse' that declares the centrality of the family in the care for older people as an unassailable African value and model could well be a key reason for the lack of specific inquiry and debate (Aboderin and Hoffman, 2012).

The disconnect between the prevailing discourse on and actual realities of long-term care for dependent older adults in SSA essentially denotes a 'lag' between evolving 'material' conditions of care and the dominant 'socio-cultural' perspectives that accompany it. This 'lag', if not challenged, will continue to impede effective debate, as well as urgently needed appropriate policy action, for mitigating caregiver strain and care inadequacies in the region (Aboderin and Hoffman, Forthcoming; Riley and Riley, 1994).

Aims and scope

Generously funded by the Marie Curie Foundation, this volume brings together the notions of space and practice in relation to care. It aims to initiate a conversation among social researchers about informal–formal/ private–public spaces and practices of care *for* SSA's vulnerable older populations.

Against the background of changing demographic and cultural trends in SSA generally, this volume also aims to emphasise heterogeneity in that ageing experiences, policies and practices are embedded in different geographies, spaces and multi-disciplinary configurations. Place and space broadly affect older people, their families and others involved in services and care. Heterogeneity in terms of enabling/ disabling environments, liveability, gender, welfare regimes, stage of the demographic transition (timing) within and across localities are increasingly being recognised by policymakers, planners, service providers and older people themselves. Through its collection of in-depth ethnographic analyses this volume proposes to show how these changes are affecting the contemporary life-worlds of SSA's older people in need of social and health care. Case studies from different regions of the continent (southern, central, eastern and western Africa) provide insights and stimulate thinking about how local and global transformations affect the ways that older people negotiate access to and/or receive social and health care within (informal) familial and/or (formal) societal contexts. In particular, it will be evident that space and place markedly affect older people's quality of life and opportunities for negotiating a good old age.

Ageing and aged African residents are the protagonists of the analyses in this volume. Who cares for them? What do they expect from care? And how are their expectations and experiences related to larger dynamics within their societies? Furthermore, how does the dominant discourse of 'the family will care' relate to realities of caregiving for older people: the extent of care needs; the care options and structures available to families; the amount, type and adequacy of the care received; the impacts on caregivers and recipients; and their own normative perceptions on who ought to provide care and why? Who takes care of older people, and where? How is this negotiated? Which institutions define older people as their clients/consumers/ target audiences? What social and institutional spaces exist where older Africans are considered as belonging to a separate social category? How did global and local histories converge to create spaces and times of vulnerability for SSA's older people, and how did this affect or contribute to resilient responses to vulnerabilities? All these questions show that there is a need for scholars of ageing research in SSA to recognise and address the current structural lag in long-term social and health care provision for dependent older people.

Van Eeuwijk (2006) indicates that, from an older person's perspective, old-age vulnerability is strongly shaped by care provision, or its lack, when in need of support. In line with Lefebvre's analysis of

3

the production of space (1991), we argue that places where care is negotiated and practised are social spaces, whether these practices are carried out by kin, professionals (nurses, doctors, healers), or 'strangers'. Spatial practices and perceptions are shaped by value judgement, the enactment of which obtains political responsibility and agency. As a consequence, spaces where care is performed acquire a political character in line with the distribution of duties, dependency and authority.

The analyses in this volume depart from similar socio-political approaches towards the concept of 'old age'. The definitions of who is 'old' and what it means 'to be old' in contemporary Africa are very much socially determined. Notions of elderliness and seniority are by no means fixed. Adeboye (2007) draws attention to the ways in which the idiom of 'old age', in the Yoruba context, has undergone significant changes since the nineteenth century – in particular through militarism, patronage, and, later on, western education and (post-) colonial governance. He argues that 'elderly authority' and status serve as metaphors that enable individuals and groups to appropriate a degree of respect, hitherto considered the prerogative of 'elders', for themselves. The idiom of 'old age' remains significant in structuring power relationships, as well as a weapon especially exploited in political contexts. Apart from this flexible idea of 'the elder', it is important to emphasise that the notion of 'elder' is also very much a social shifter. This concept of the 'social shifter' is inspired by Durham (2000), who uses it in the context of youth in Africa. A shifter is a linguistic category. A deictic or indexical term (like 'I', 'here' or 'now') acts as a shifter and works not through absolute referentiality to a fixed context but connects the speaker to a relational, or indexical, context. Linguistic shifters thus draw out the metalinguistic features of the conversation. Durham (2000, 116) argues that the use of 'youth' (but we could say the same for 'elderly/older people') evokes a 'social landscape of power, rights, expectations and relationships – indexing both themselves and the topology of that social landscape'. Physical/chronological old age notwithstanding, it is one's position within social networks that defines one as an 'elder/grand/big person' or as a 'petit/small person'. Such relative approaches towards 'old age' render the study of ageing in Africa particularly challenging, and must be included in any examination of 'elderly' life-worlds in Africa and the diasporas, as these relative positions also carry responsibilities and rights.

To this end, the specific directions pursued in this volume of eight contributions include: sound grounded investigations of private and public perspectives and rationales regarding the role of familial/formal care; an explicit engagement with existing policy and public debates and frameworks concerning the culture of care; and the conceptual development of perspectives dealing with how formal care provision can be reconciled with local values of respect for older people and family obligations.

Four interrelating spaces are explored in this book's contributions: the first presents an exploration of contemporary care relationships within and across generations; the second focuses on tensions in the actual care management of older people among individuals, families, societies and the state; third, the rural/urban nexus is explored in relation to care for older people; and fourth, care is envisaged as a negotiated commodity. The volume's cross-cutting aims are therefore to

- examine the extent to which present discourses and policy agendas are reflective of emergent insights on the realities of care in SSA;
- identify implications for further research and debate, as well as policy and programmatic interventions.

The issue of social and health care for older people in SSA moreover cuts across a wide range of domains (family, intergenerational, health, liveability, development, poverty, sense of place, social protection, provision of services and so on) increasingly demanding the attention of social and health practitioners, policy makers and scholars alike. This volume's contribution chiefly lies in the fact that contemporary long-term care management for older people in SSA is under-researched and an increasingly conceptual/policy/practice dilemma. The more original contribution, however, is that this volume attempts to face up to the existing lag, namely how the ideal of the African family relates to the realities of inter- and intra-generational relations and support in the region. To this end the contributions in this volume:

- offer original ethnographic data from southern, central, eastern and western Africa;
- critically identify 'new' spaces of care;
- describe new dynamics in the practices of care (for example, older people caring for other older people; retirement homes);
- study 'care' as a negotiated commodity;
- provide conceptual, policy and programmatic inferences.

Themes: spaces of care and care practices

More specifically the interrelated notions of spaces and practices of care are highlighted in greater detail:

The production of spaces of care

Attention to the production of spaces of care is critical to the study of older people's life-worlds. Place emerges as an important matter of concern in the ageing process (see Obrist, Chapter Four). Questions like 'who will take care of me when I become immobile or frail?' push many people to reflect on their relationships with their kin and kith. Older people's mobility, and incremental immobility once the body starts to slow down, makes them increasingly aware of the availability, or unavailability, of care opportunities in a given environment. Various places are discussed in the next chapters: the house; the neighbourhood; the hospital; the home of a healer; the retirement home. Although these are all places, they are not always spaces of care. It is the performance of care activities, specifically, that transforms these places into spaces of care. Sheltering and providing accommodation are among various broad care activities. In his ethnography of care among Botswana's Christian believers in the midst of the AIDS crisis, Klaits (2010, 101) indicates that housing (sheltering people) relates to love and care (just as it may incite jealousy and scorn). As Klaits (2010, 120) indicates in terms of social relationships and physical wellbeing: where you are, affects who you are. For older people, security does not only depend on having offspring, but also, and probably most importantly, on the 'children's willingness to...stay with or build for them' (Klaits, 2010, 87). Klaits observes that his informants pay a great deal of attention to the movement of people, the various places (towns, villages, fields, cattle posts) and the sets of people among whom they move over time, as well as how these movements relate to the care, love, scorn and jealousy for people in particular places. Emotions and affects circulate within these spaces, along with obligations and responsibilities. Fears and anxieties stimulate older people to move or be moved.

The home is the primary space of care for older people in all the locales studied in this book. The home is often taken as synonymous with 'the family', which could be a spouse and/or offspring (classificatory children and grandchildren included). In most instances the family as the first space of care is so self-evident that older people do not even mention family members as caregivers (see Freeman, Chapter Five). Yet in different contexts *home* is not always constituted by the same categories. While Obrist (Chapter Four) found that *home* refers to the physical structures that her various respondents in Tanzania built or bought, Van Eeuwijk (Chapter Three) shows that *home* can also be constituted of other categories: increasingly siblings or other family members join the household of an older person in need of care as co-residents; or care activities are provided by people with whom the older person does not necessarily share a living space, for example relatives living abroad send money home for medical costs; or relatives come to visit a particular older person. Even in these instances the (extended) family is expected to remain the first social space of care. In Tanzania Obrist notes embarrassment or shame when people have recourse to neighbours or others.

The absence or presence of support leads people to move older people in need of care around; alternatively the older people themselves choose to move around. This spatial flux transcends the assumption that older people are static and stuck. Apart from the presence of a caregiver, the economic capacities of the hosting (caring) family unit also determine where an older person in need of care can be housed. Hoffman (Chapter Seven) mentions a hierarchy of needs, which his South African participants laid bare. He found that the needs of the immediate family (in contrast to the extended family) and of the younger generations are prioritised. Pype (Chapter Two) observes similar issues with the childless widows of polygamous men. These women could be taken care of by a co-wife's children as long as that particular co-wife was alive, or as long as there was extra money and space available to house her. However, as soon as any of these securitising criteria disappear, the elderly widow is the first to be neglected and even chased out of the compound.

There is variation in expectations regarding which particular kin is supposed to take care of a needy older person: whereas Van Eeuwijk states that in Tanzania it is ideally the offspring that support and help their older people, Freeman found that in rural Malawi, elder-to-elder care (usually provided by an elderly co-spouse) is the norm. Nonetheless, societies are continuously undergoing change, and Van Eeuwijk found that the majority of care arrangements actually point to intra-generational care where capable older people care for needy elderly. A similar observation has been made for South Africa (see Hoffman, Chapter Seven).

None of this suggests that care is a taken-for-granted performance of the family. There are several reasons. First and foremost, there is the economy of care. Some authors argue that 'family care is in crisis' (see Van der Geest, 1997; 2002; Aboderin, 2006). Care is something in which people must invest during their lifetimes. Those who have not sufficiently invested in relationships with others who might later care for them cannot expect anything from others. Thus, the social space of care does not emerge out of the blue; rather, it is the outcome of many years of efforts, of attention, contribution and support. The wise person thinks about those who will be able to feed and house him/her in the not-so-distant future. This idea of reciprocity that undergirds, in various chapters, the performance of care is gradually giving way to the acceptance of the professionalisation of care. Van Eeuwijk shows how, in Tanzania, various non-kin support groups (ethnic-related, religious, state and NGO-led) provide care for older people. Demographic changes can also contribute to this shift towards non-kin care.

Van der Geest (Chapter One) explicitly mentions the fact that as people become older, the focus is more and more on the core family instead of the extended family. Avoidance rules can also shape the moral expectations of the family as the immediate space of care. Obrist (Chapter Four) observes that avoidance rules based on gender and generation prohibit daughters from performing the most intimate activities of care (washing the bodies and clothes of elderly relatives); while in Kinshasa, rules forbidding sons-in-law from seeing their mothers-in-law naked and vice-versa, impelled some women to move to retirement homes. Yet, older people themselves sometimes make it impossible for their own offspring to take care of them. For example, in Kinshasa again, some older people quarrelled with their children and decided to no longer live with them, thus moving to a retirement home. Freeman, by contrast, notes that her research participants in rural Malawi held strongly to the idea of the adult as an autonomous self-sufficient person who endeavoured to remain independent as long as possible. Here, 'bad old age' means not being able to care for oneself. Similar ideas about not wanting to be a burden to their offspring arise elsewhere as well, pushing elderly people to remain independent as long as possible.

Finally, changing opinions about who should care for whom and where are evolving, and also increasingly influencing the operationalisation of care. Especially in South Africa, younger generations see institutional care as viable (Hoffman, Chapter Seven). While in Tanzania, as already mentioned, non-kin groups also perform the tasks of care (Van Eeuwijk, Chapter Three). Van der Geest (Chapter One) begins his analysis on Ghanaian care practices with a reflection from one of his research participants, who warmed to the idea of being housed in a retirement home and thus being among peers. However, that same respondent pointed at the Ghanaian state – and especially at its incompetence in carrying out the tasks of a public service provider – as the reason he was not yet living in that retirement facility.

Interestingly, the 'ideal of the family taking care of older people' appears time and again in the discourses of retirement home residents; those older people who are cared for by non-kin still usually try to excuse their own families (see Hoffman, Chapter Seven and Pype, Chapter Two), thus illustrating that the family's reputation remains something older people want to protect. Yet the mere fact that they are cared for outside the kin space questions the relatives' possibilities or desire to care for them. In contesting critiques that it lacks initiative in this domain, the Ghanaian state also purchases the moral obligation of the 'African family' as the primary care provider. Some countries pay retirement pensions to older people, yet this goes hand in hand with a particular politics. In Kinshasa, it has been observed that people keep older people in their homes because of the pension some receive every three months. The pension thus becomes a voucher for care within the family.

Various contributors raise the issue of paid care. As mentioned earlier Obrist (Chapter Four), shows that her research participants indicated experiencing shame when having to request assistance from neighbours. However, this feeling was absent in the case of paid help. Van der Geest refers to Dsane's research (2013) in Ghana where middle-class and well-to-do families utilise external facilities, such as daycare centres and retirement homes, as appropriate spaces for their ageing kin. There are thus indications that outsourcing becomes an increasingly accepted reality. Still, there is an exchange, a reciprocity, at work. It manifests as economic capital, in paying others to perform care for older family members. It does not contradict the debt logic (Marie, 2000) between generations; rather, it has simply added intermediaries in the performance of care. In a number of African cities, NGOs are increasingly discovering the life-worlds of older people as interesting social spaces; and some older people are also eagerly taking advantage of these new spaces (windows) of opportunity (see Van Eeuwijk, Chapter Three).

The city as such is another spatial category that very much determines people's expectations and actual practices of care. Overall, urban contexts provide new modes of self-definition and social interaction. This also plays out in the semantic and political fields of generations, youth and old age. When Pype first presented her research project on old age to colleagues at the University of Kinshasa, two issues came to the fore: colleagues emphasised the role of material culture in the establishment of elders' authority and the stigmatisation of older people in the city. They argued that respect for, but also fear of, older people depend a great deal on the *attributes* older people possess. However, some argued that 'the objects of authority and power that old people possess in the village, are no longer used in the city'. In addition, when they conducted their own surveys in Kinshasa, they noticed that people were afraid of giving their age for fear of being treated as an 'old person'. This fear is understandable. The social positioning of elders in urban contexts is precarious, and there is a wide gap between the ideal and the actual ways in which 'old people' are regarded.

Neglect, or the absence of one or more activities related to care, is a recurrent topic in the chapters. Neglect becomes first and foremost visible in the elder's body, yet also speaks to the older person's social context. As De Klerk states in Chapter Six, a well-cared-for body in an elderly person is an indication that all is well in the family. Impoverished individuals who go hungry, whose clothes are left unwashed for days, and whose wounds are not cleaned, are shut off from basic care services. Such conditions literally reveal the absence of family – the supposed first space of care. In the Kinois (Kinshasa's inhabitants) context, neighbourhood Christians are the ones conveying this lack of care to the church, and, if necessary, to state agents (Chapter Three). There are various reasons for the absence of care within the family, but lack of offspring, economic deprivation and out-migration are the main vectors that render older people vulnerable and excluded from immediate care provision. Interestingly, several chapters also point to the responsibility of the elders themselves when they are neglected by kin. As De Klerk shows, some have made mistakes in the past by not investing enough in individuals who could care for them in later years. In the Kinois context, Pype shows that some elderly men decide to break all ties with their offspring, and this is most manifestly reflected in moving out of the house and moving into a retirement home.

It is precisely this absence of good care that pushes older people to be mobile. De Klerk describes the trajectory of an elderly woman who chooses to move back to the village after having a falling out with her granddaughter. Her decision in turn led to new conflicts within the family. So while older people's mobility (often shaped by the absence or presence of care) is informed by the (extended) family, it also transforms the dynamics within the family. When that same Tanzanian woman was beaten in the village, her grandson decided to call her back to the city. Similar tensions between absence/presence of care and older people's movements (or lack thereof) colour all dynamics and analyses in this volume.

Practices

The volume is furthermore inscribed within practice theory – exploring ways in which social subjects are produced through practice, and how they, in turn, create their worlds via practice. The contributors' analyses are close to Ortner's correction of practice theory (2006), where she tries to come to terms with the fact that people are born within a society governed by social structures but at the same time can also claim agency and decide not to comply with given norms and ideals, or else modify them. In this sense, we come to a theoretical focus that accepts the influence, of on the one hand, 'tradition', 'state prescriptions', and family obligations for caregiving, while on the other hand her analysis also allows for those who – whether deliberately or not – position themselves outside of normative orders and participate in emerging registers of concern, aid and assistance. Care provision in contemporary Africa is embedded within political, economic and societal transformations in the different societies under consideration. Careful ethnographic analysis is needed to tease out all the variations in care provision for older people, in different locales, in order to better understand who is experiencing care, and how. Who is controlling care provision, and how does this happen? All the chapters in this volume, therefore, delineate ways in which practices of care are shaped by expectations – often deduced from norms – and actual experiences – informed by the quotidian, which itself relies on contingency and uncertainty (Cooper and Pratten, 2015).

This volume's attention to practices includes first and foremost a focus on those social categories that provide care services. Its chapters show that an ever more diversified group of caregivers is emerging. It is no longer merely children and grandchildren who are involved in caregiving. Rather, elderly people also wash, monitor, cook for and feed fellow older people (Van Eeuwijk, Chapter Three); strangers, that is, people unrelated to older people, also take on several caring activities. As Pype shows, in the Kinois context, bringing clothes and food to retirement homes and keeping older people company – while hardly intervening in their private lives – are practices enacted by entrepreneurs, who, with intentions of turning bad money into good, take on these roles. While these strangers only appear at retirement homes irregularly, the nurses, cleaners and social workers hired by the state or by NGOs constitute another category of unrelated individuals who, in exchange for a salary, take on the task of helping needy older people. In addition, in certain contexts, children and grandchildren can also provide care 'from a distance'. Relatives living in the diaspora count it among their responsibilities to ensure that their ageing parents are well cared for. Although physically absent, they attempt to influence their older relatives' wellbeing by having a say about where their relatives should be housed; by sending money to them and their caregivers, who are very often (classificatory) siblings of those in the diaspora; by sending commodities (for example, mobile phones (see Pype, 2016), but also medicine and clothes) to their older relatives; by speaking to them over the phone; and, albeit rarely, by moving them abroad.

Van der Geest (2002, 9–17) describes the following care activities, according to his rural Akan informants: feeding, bathing, clothing, helping older people to use the toilet, providing money, providing company, and organising a suitable funeral. Following this definition, it becomes clear that practices of care extend beyond an immediate attention to primary needs. Rather, older people who prepare for their old age by investing in ties with individuals who, they hope, will care for them, or by moving to another place where they think they will be less of a burden to others, and by preparing their deaths and funerals, perform actions that influence the forms and duration of care. In the Kinois context, once again, Pype learned from several research participants that they participated in ristournes (rotating saving schemes) to help them collect money for their funerals. Such actions would ensure a good funeral. Instead of counting on the financial capacities of their relatives (children included), which are never assured, these elderly preferred investing their own money in a good (expensive) funeral. Many Kinois become nervous if they do not yet own a house by their 40s or 50s. Such fears express the anticipation of a lack of hospitality from relatives. Similar anxieties regarding lack of space can be observed in Tanzania, where landholding and endowing are crucial practices in guaranteeing care in old age (De Klerk, Chapter Six).

A number of authors in this volume reflect on the body. First, caregiving is indeed an embodied practice, especially because washing, clothing, feeding and providing medical treatment to elderly people are activities that can require a great deal of strength from caregivers. However, the main focus in these chapters is on the body of the care-receiver. Primary activities of care ensures the physical survival of the older person. Second, growing old is also very much a bodily process and the taken-for-granted reciprocity between generations resides, as Freeman shows, sometimes literally in the blood and/or the semen. As lineage belonging is often physically mediated (as in motherhood), along come responsibilities and obligations towards people with whom 'one shares blood'.

A chronological orientation of chapters in this volume

More specifically, the volume kicks off with the provocative question by Van der Geest in Chapter One, namely 'Will families in Ghana continue to care for older people?' Ghanaian politicians and moral authorities insist that care for older people is and must remain a family responsibility. They sharply criticise the use of old people's homes and other care institutions in high-income 'western' countries. This chapter presents a case study of care of older people in order to explore the future feasibility of keeping older people in their homes, with their children and grandchildren. The study is based in Kwahu, where care for older people is indeed largely carried out by family members, but where cracks in the traditional system have begun to appear in the complaints of older people about loneliness and lack of respect. The question is whether economic growth and improvement of medical care, with its ensuing lengthening of life, will eventually lead to 'western' conditions in Ghana. Given the possibility that future generations of Ghanaians may become even more mobile, have fewer children, live increasingly in nuclear families and grow older, Van der Geest hypothesises that families will find it increasingly challenging to provide good care for their ageing parents and will look for new care alternatives.

Van der Geest is followed by Pype's contribution (Chapter Two), in which she considers an alternative care option, namely the retirement home in a post-colonial setting as a space between the family, the state and the church. Most of these retirement homes in Kinshasa were created during colonial times and are physical reminders of western spatial politics of care provision for older people. Nowadays, retirement homes constitute knots of various intentionalities: Christian clergy, state functionaries, local benefactors and (to a lesser extent) foreign NGO workers. Her chapter provides an analysis of interviews with the 'indigents' (indigent people), as the residents of Kinshasa's retirement homes are known. Among her points of foci are the various social spaces these older people traversed before arriving at the retirement home. This material allows us to identify 'ideal' and 'actual' practices of caretaking of older people in a post-colonial setting. While clichés about *African* solidarity within the family thrive among Kinois, Kinshasa's older people experience various kinds of social exclusion, ranging from being accused of witchcraft to having become a financial burden for their relatives, and experience physical exclusion from the family home due to illness, handicap, or merely fatigue, as well as cultural taboos. This material, obtained via observation and personal narratives, is further complemented with data collected during interviews with state officials (Ministry of Social Affairs, urban authorities for older people, national agencies for the retired and retirement home personnel), church leaders, older people living among kin, relatives of 'indigents', and *donateurs* (benefactors donating money, medicine, clothes, food, wheelchairs and the like to residents of retirement homes).

Van Eeuwijk's contribution explores the intergenerational/intra-generational care nexus in rural and urban Tanzania (Chapter Three). This chapter about care *within* generations offers an immediate alternative to the more conventional care contract *between* younger and older generations, as extensively explored in Aboderin's (2006) book *Intergenerational support and old age in Africa*. While older people acting as caregivers for HIV/AIDS orphans is a well-documented phenomenon in Tanzania, a surprisingly high number of older people were found to act as primary caregivers for other older people in need of some kind of support. They provide care to members of their own generation (intra-generational care arrangements) or to members of their parent's generation (intergenerational). The most frequent care arrangement, that of an older wife taking care of her aged husband, further shows the gendered nature of care. Care of older people provided by aged people is regarded as an implicit failure of intergenerational kin obligations and its corresponding negotiations – care provision by older people is believed to go against the convention of 'filial duty'. However, at critical health moments where physical, emotional, financial, and medical support are urgently needed, close family members (for example, children, grandchildren and/or siblings) often join the care arrangements and assist the older care provider. This 'kinning by care' is not only consistent with the normative principles of care provision; it also represents to some degree the capability of older caregivers to mobilise social networks for needed care support. Additionally, non-kin care of older people provided by, for instance, religious groups, widows' clubs, or NGOs is gaining prominence in Tanzania – and in most cases these institutions' caregiving members are themselves older people (and mostly women). Despite its mostly supportive and complementary nature this 'care work' by older people is increasingly transforming care into both a commodity (for example, profit and profession) and a 'gatekeeping' function.

Obrist (Chapter Four) straddles the spaces and practices of living and care arrangements for frail older people in rural and urban Tanzania. Based on ethnographic case studies in diverse contexts of coastal Tanzania, her chapter explores the meanings of frailty and associated care arrangements for and by older people. Older men and women often complain about loss of strength, weight loss, limited physical activity, lack of endurance and fatigue. While many of them attributed these bodily experiences to advanced stages of ageing, others saw their causes in a specific disease, an injury, or a more general malaise. What practical and social implications do these experiences of frailty have for daily living arrangements? Do other people step in to provide special care, and if so, who gives what kind of care, and when? How do kinship, gender and generation intersect in care arrangements? What kinds of spaces are created by diverse arrangements? Living and care arrangements often did not correspond. Common modalities included somebody in the same house providing care, somebody coming in to provide care, or older people being moved nearer to care providers. Those engaged in day-to-day practical and emotional care were mostly women linked to the frail elderly through extended family relations. Men as husbands, brothers and sons were also involved in certain forms of practical and emotional care, but more often they were responsible for organising financial, logistical and administrative support, especially when professional care was needed. A focus on *doing care* for frail older people reveals that all care is clearly embedded in broader fields of social practice.

Chapter Five, which draws on sociological and social psychological theories of identity in order to analyse the ethnographic data presented, centres on care as an embodied practice. Along with contributions by Obrist (Chapter Four) and De Klerk (Chapter Six), Freeman argues that incorporating the body and its meanings into the study of care in Africa enriches explorations of how care is experienced, and could lead to more sensitive representations of care and ageing in social policy and practice. Set in a poor, subsistence agriculture, region of Malawi and drawing on interviews with men and women aged between 50 and 100, Freeman discusses how older people felt about receiving care. In their narratives, expectations of care and attitudes towards receiving care offer understandings of what it means to be old, even as identities are challenged and preserved. While the receipt of day-to-day assistance from those able to provide it could be incorporated into older people's positive age-related identity scripts, receipt of care from those who could not easily provide it, or when given in response to vulnerability, were framed with reference to overwhelmingly negative understandings of old age, which, in turn, presented a challenge to older men and women's core identities as 'adults'. Older people's emphasis on self-care and reciprocal exchanges of care could thus be considered as a strategy for maintaining positive 'adult' identities. In this discussion, the construction of an *African* group identity where 'the family will care' is furthermore distorted. This ideal appears to have little salience for older men and women in rural Malawi. They present expectations of care that are heavily dependent on individual circumstances and understandings of care.

De Klerk (Chapter Six) explores the intimacy of the physicality of care. In northwest Tanzania, the absence of institutional forms of old-age care, and the poor implementation of old-age care policies in health facilities, place care firmly in the domain of the family. The presence of AIDS over the past 25 years and the movement of young adults to cities, have profoundly changed these social forms of old-age care, creating care relations and care expectations around old-age care that are new and contested. At the same time new technologies are introducing novel forms of old-age care: mobile technology brings migrated children closer, and a health programme of a local NGO has, since 2010, increasingly introduced exercise classes to help older people become more self-reliant, thereby influencing ideas around family care for older people. Older people emphasise the need for a strong body, as an able body is an essential element in the consolidation of social and family relations in this uncertain environment; yet the abilities of ageing bodies are also inherently uncertain. To overcome the limitations of their ageing bodies, the importance of physical strength to engage in these family relations is increasingly important, especially for older women. This chapter focuses particularly on how older women increasingly refer to their fragile bodies in relation to obtaining old-age care, not just to lament the loss of care, but also to find subtle ways of presenting their aged bodies for obtaining care.

In Chapter Seven, the last of the case studies, Hoffman explores the moral space in which care is negotiated in the context of poverty and HIV/AIDS in South Africa. Around 6 million people in South Africa live with HIV/AIDS. Of the estimated 1.2 million children orphaned by AIDS, approximately 60 per cent live in grandparent-headed multi-generational families where grandmothers in particular act as surrogate parents. They often also simultaneously care for HIV-positive adult children. Through a generational sequential approach based on 58 narratives from 20 multi-generational networks in Mpumalanga (South Africa), this contribution explores the complex nature of the relationship between different generations in the context of poverty and HIV/AIDS, where there is mainly downward support. The findings strongly indicate that both older and younger generations recognise the collective ideal of reciprocal support. The respective generations, however, differ in their views for implementing this ideal. Older carers (mainly women) contribute support despite the impact of context –

their motivation being that younger generations should always enjoy precedence. Younger generations, for their part, argue that support to older generations is mediated by context: they are influenced by competing priorities for their time and resources, often leaving older generations without adequate support. Younger generations, moreover, increasingly perceive institutional care as a viable option. The moral space between the perceived normative ideal and the pragmatics of the moment provides a scope of negotiation to regenerate or contest the care relationship. However, these differential obligations and priorities often leave older carers particularly vulnerable in terms of their own future care outcomes.

The volume concludes with an extensive afterword in which Baart draws on the preceding cases and discourses (Chapters One to Seven) in order to provide a conceptual framework – a starting point at least to conceptualise contemporary care *for* older people in SSA. This chapter endeavours to move beyond what Hagestad and Dannefer (2001) describe as the microfication of social research on ageing: an analytical trend that results in an over-emphasis of micro-interactions between individuals, with the result that macro-phenomena like social institutions, cohesion, conflict, norms and values become invisible. A close analysis of personal accounts and situated meaning-making does not necessarily have to equal methodological microfication if explicit, rigorous, reflexive and transparent descriptions of samples, contexts and processes are considered. These first level narratives, grounded in people's lived experiences, however, lead to a core SSA story beyond microfication. Such a core story implies neither uniformity in participants' experiences nor a predictable general sequential pattern, but offers broad cross-cutting storylines, as presented by Baart on the basis of his discourse analysis of the preceding chapters. In order to develop such a core story as starting point, Baart's immediate aim is to offer a conceptual next step to illustrate how to utilise discourse analysis to better understand the challenge of long-term care for older people in SSA, and possible interventions.

Directions for further research

An edited volume such as this one has its limitations, and one obvious lacuna concerns care across transnational spaces and how this affects practices. More work is also needed on virtual spaces, especially in view of the deep penetration of mobile phone technology in SSA, and how care practices could be affected in the near future.

It is anticipated that this volume, complementary to the other volumes published over nearly two decades (see Apt, 1996; Makoni and Stroeken, 2002; Aboderin, 2006; Cole and Durham, 2007; Cohen and Menken, 2006; Alber et al, 2008; Maharaj, 2012), will invigorate research, as well as relevant policy and programmatic interventions in long-term care provision for dependent older people in SSA, recognising and addressing the current structural lag. Future empirical research and critical academic discourse can play important roles in this regard. Specific directions to be pursued to this end include more

1. explicit engagement with existing policy, and public debates and frameworks on the culture of care;
2. large-scale research to establish and quantify the impacts (health, social, economic) of current informal care arrangements;
3. sound grounded investigation of public perspectives, rationales on the role of formal care;
4. conceptual development, possibly drawing on parallel experiences in Asian societies, of perspectives on how formal care provision can be reconciled with values of respect for older people and family obligations in Africa and its diasporas.

References

Aboderin, I, 2006, *Intergenerational support and old age in Africa*, London: Transaction Publishers

Aboderin, I, Hoffman, J, 2012, Care for older adults in Sub-Saharan Africa: Discourses and realities of family solidarity, invited Presidential Symposium: *Taking care? Global discourses on intergenerational relationships and Family support*, 65th Annual Scientific Meeting, Gerontological Society of America (GSA), 14–18 November, San Diego, USA

Aboderin, I, Hoffman, J, Forthcoming, Policy on long term care for older people in Sub-Saharan Africa: confronting a structural lag, *Journal of Cross-Cultural Gerontology*

Adeboye, O, 2007, The changing conception of elderhood in Ibadan, 1830–2000, *Nordic Journal of African Studies* 16, 2, 261–78

Alber, E, Van der Geest, S, Whyte, SR (eds), 2008, *Generations in Africa: Connections and conflicts*, Münster: LIT Verlag

Apt, N, 1996, *Coping with old age in a changing Africa: Social change and the elderly Ghanaian*, Aldershot: Avebury

Ardington, C, Case, A, Islam, M, Lam, D, Leibbrandt, M, Menendez, A, Olgiatia, A, 2010, The impact of AIDS on intergenerational support in South Africa: Evidence from the Cape Area panel study, *Research on Aging* 32, 1, 97–121

Barrientos, A, Ferreira, M, Gorman, M, Heslop, A, Legido-Quigley, H, Lloyd-Sherlock, P, Møller, V, Saboia, J, Werneck, MLT, 2003, *Non-contributory pensions and poverty prevention: A comparative study of South Africa and Brazil*, London: HelpAge International and Institute for Development Policy and Management

Cassim, B, Rauff, S, McIntyre, J, Van der Pas, S, Deeg, D, 2012, The impact of cognitive impairment on care received and well-being in older South Africans, *1st IAGG Africa Region Congress on Gerontology and Geriatrics*, 17–20 October, Cape Town, South Africa

Cohen, B, Menken, J (eds), 2006, *Aging in sub-Saharan Africa: Recommendations for furthering research*, Washington, DC: The National Academies Press

Cole, J, Durham, D (eds), 2007, *Generations and globalization: Youth, age, and family in the new world economy*, Bloomington, IN: Indiana University Press

Cooper, E, Pratten, D (eds), 2015, *Ethnographies of uncertainty in Africa*, London: Palgrave MacMillan

Dsane, S, 2013, Can 'strangers' provide care for frail older people in Ga families?, Draft paper, presented at the international conference 'Revisiting the first international congress of Africanists in a globalised world', 24–26 October, Institute of African Studies, University of Ghana

Durham, D, 2000, Youth and the social imagination in Africa: Introduction to parts 1 and 2, *Anthropological Quarterly* 73, 3, 113–20

Hagestad, GO, Dannefer, D, 2001, Concepts and theories of aging: Beyond micro-fication in social sciences approaches, in RH Binstock, L George (eds) *Handbook of aging and social sciences*, pp 3–21, San Diego, CA: Academic

Klaits, F, 2010, *Death in a church of life: Moral passion during Botswana's time of aids*, Berkeley, CA: University of California Press

Lefebvre, H, 1991, *The production of space*, translated by D Nicholson-Smith, Oxford: Blackwell

Madhavan, S, 2004, Fosterage patterns in the age of AIDS: Continuity and change, *Social Science and Medicine* 58, 1443–54

Maharaj, P (ed), 2012, *Aging and health in Africa*, New York: Springer

Makoni, S, Stroeken, K, 2002, *Ageing in Africa: Linguistic and anthropological approaches*, Farnham: Ashgate

Marie, A, 2000, Individualization strategies among city dwellers in contemporary Africa: Balancing the shortcomings of community solidarity and the individualism of the struggle for survival, *International Review of Social History* 11, 45, 37–57

Ortner, S, 2006, *Anthropology and social theory: Culture, power, and the acting subject*, Durham, NC: Duke University Press

Phaswana-Mafuya, N, Peltzer, K, Chirinda, W, Kose, Z, Hoosain, E, Ramlagan, S, Tabane, C, Davids, AS, 2012, Health status of older South Africans: Evidence from SAGE, *1st IAGG Africa Region Conference on Gerontology and Geriatrics*, 17–20 October, Cape Town, South Africa

Pype, K, 2016, Brokers of belonging: Elders and intermediaries in Kinshasa's mobile phone culture, in W Mano, W Willems (eds) *Everyday media culture in Africa: Audiences and users*, London: Routledge. (In press)

Riley, MW, Riley, JW, 1994, Structural lag: Past and future, in MW Riley, RL Khan, A Foner (eds) *Age and structural lag: Society's failure to find meaningful opportunities in work, family and leisure*, pp 15–36, New York: Wiley

Roser, M, 2015, Life expectancy, published online at OurWorldInData.org, http://ourworldindata.org/data/population-growth-vital-statistics/life-expectancy/

UNPD (United Nations Population Division), 2012, *World population prospects: The 2010 revision*, New York: UNPD, http://esa.un.org/unpp/

Van der Geest, S, 1997, Money and respect: The changing value of old age in rural Ghana, *Africa: Journal of the International African Institute* 76, 4, 534–59

Van der Geest, S, 2002, Respect and reciprocity: Care of elderly people in rural Ghana, *Journal of Cross-Cultural Gerontology* 17, 3–31

Van Eeuwijk, P, 2006, Old-age vulnerability, ill-health and care support in urban areas of Indonesia, *Ageing and Society*, 26, 61–80

Will families in Ghana continue to care for older people? Logic and contradiction in policy

Sjaak van der Geest

Introduction

During conversations with older (and younger) people in Kwahu–Tafo, a rural town in southern Ghana, I sometimes brought up the topic of old people's homes as they exist in my own country, the Netherlands. The older people then asked what those homes looked like and I described them in as neutral terms as possible. Some of the older people rejected the idea of handing over the care of older relatives to 'strangers' but surprisingly most reacted positively, even enthusiastically. One older man, living without any relatives in his own house, responded:

> That would be very, very good for Ghana. I for one if I had been taken to an institution to care for me, I would be happy. Because, when I get there, I will meet my classmates and friends. [Here] in the house, you will always find me alone, if my wife is not around. There will be no wife and so your partners [other residents] will be your 'wife' and everything. You will take the old people as your mates…If my wife is not strong and I feel lonely, I will prefer to go there. You are comforted…some happiness, games, crack jokes, and so on. You won't remember anything [you won't worry about anything]. But when you are alone, you will think [be troubled] all the time. If you are properly fed, breakfast, lunch and dinner, you won't feel anything.

Often, however, when the discussion continued, doubts began to arise: Ghana was too poor to run such homes for older people. Moreover, the homes would be overcrowded in no time as everybody would rush to live there. So, old people's homes did not seem a realistic option for a country like Ghana, however attractive they might seem to be.

This chapter explores what the future may hold for older people in Ghana in this era of rapid globalisation. I will first present a rural ethnographic case study of how older people are currently cared for. Next I will look at Ghanaian policy on the welfare of older people and a few attempts to find solutions for the present challenges in the care for older people due to decreasing family support, migration and increasing longevity. Finally I will draw some cautious conclusions or rather raise questions about the future of care for older people in Ghana.

Ageing and care in Kwahu-Tafo

Between 1994 and 2006 I did anthropological research about experiences of growing old and receiving care in the rural town of Kwahu-Tafo, in the Eastern Region of Ghana. The research consisted mainly of open interviews or conversations with 35 older people. All conversations were recorded and transcribed. In addition, I paid short visits that gave me an idea of the daily life of the older people. I talked to relatives, friends and acquaintances, trying in this way to form a picture of how their condition had developed into what it was. Furthermore, I tried to take part in various activities of older people. I joined some of them who were still active on their farms, I sat and conversed with them in front of their houses or in the palm wine bars, I went with them to church and attended funerals where the older people played an important role. Another part of the study consisted of (informal) 'focus group discussions' with eight to twenty people on various issues related to ageing. These discussions were also recorded and transcribed. During most conversations a co-researcher accompanied me to help with the language. Afterwards the co-researchers also discussed the contents of the conversations with me, adding their own views. The sharing of research activities is expressed by the term 'we' throughout this case study.

The study began with general questions: What does it mean to be old? How do older people view themselves? How do others see them? How are they cared for when they need help? What has changed in recent decades for them? From these general questions specific issues emerged that the older people themselves and people in their environment brought up during the discussions. These issues led to new questions and insights about, for example, respect, wisdom, witchcraft, money, building a house, and sexuality. This chapter concentrates on two such issues, namely loneliness and quality of care. But first a few words about reciprocity, because reciprocity is what care of older people depends on, as was repeatedly emphasised.

Reciprocity

The conversations and observations showed that the people in Kwahu-Tafo find that parents who really cared for their children (when they were young) are entitled to receive good care from their children when they have grown old. If they have not been good parents they forfeit that right. As one old cocoa farmer said, 'I am old but very happy because I looked after my children and now they are feeding me... Nothing worries me.' We asked another older person why in some houses, there are old people who look miserable and neglected. He replied: 'If you lay a good foundation, you will reap the results, but if you failed to look after the people around you, they won't spend their money on you when you are old. Such miserable, old people are those who failed to work hard in their youth.' A young woman declared that she would, to the best of her ability, look after her old mother, who had worked hard for her, but that she would not care at all for her old father since the man had done nothing for her when she was a child.

Migration and children's long-term absence, which have changed so much in the life of the town would, however, not affect the 'golden rule' of reciprocity as was repeatedly claimed. One woman said: 'If the parents looked well after their children, no matter what will happen, the children will also care for their parents. Even if the children have travelled outside the town or outside Ghana, they will remit their parents. All depends on the care the parents gave to the children in their early years.'[1]

That does not mean, however, that this is always the case. Sometimes children are simply not able to provide proper care. Isabella Aboderin (2006) made similar observations in her study of older people in the urban environment of the capital Accra. In some other cases, parents who do not 'deserve' it do receive good care.

Divorce and separation, common phenomena at advanced age, should also be seen in the light of reciprocity. A woman may find that her husband invested insufficiently in his marriage and so she feels no obligation towards him when he becomes dependent. He has given very little during his active life and will give her nothing in the years to come. That unattractive prospect may make her decide to leave him and return to her own relatives. She will look for security from her children and her family of birth (abusua).

Loneliness among older people

In popular language, having lived for a long time is almost tantamount to being wise.[2] The old person has seen a lot of things; he has gained an understanding of how things work and has learned how to prevent misfortune. Such knowledge is more effective than physical strength. Old people take pleasure in stressing that point all the time: the youth depend on them because of their wisdom.

The most precious company to an older person is, as one older person said, that of a young person who comes to you and asks for advice. That type of visit is a true recognition of the older person's wisdom and a convincing expression of respect. There is no greater pleasure for an older person than having such company, but there is also no greater disappointment than having none of it. This brings us to the common experience of loneliness.

Providing company to older people, especially to those who are not able to leave the house, constitutes an important aspect of care, which may have a profound effect on the older person's wellbeing. But the picture is diverse and ambiguous. During conversations an old person sometimes stressed their loneliness and boredom but on another occasion when we found the same person in another mood, they would boast about their social importance by claiming that many people visited them.

Our tentative conclusion about the older people whom we interviewed was that those who were most dependent on others for company were most likely not to get that company. Older people who were mobile and strong were able to go out and visit their friends. But those who could not leave the house and had to wait until others visited them complained that people had forgotten about them. They hardly had any visitors to receive. The claim that older people were respected because of their knowledge of tradition and wisdom and that they were consulted for advice was not supported by our findings. The interviews and observations rather suggested that the present generation was hardly interested in the knowledge of the older generation. That knowledge had become redundant and/or irrelevant to them. What they needed to know to succeed in life in this time of globalisation was not something stored in older people's memories.

Becoming dependent is a downward spiral. Those who don't go out gradually lose their social importance and become less and less interesting to visit. Being cut off from the information network that spreads through the community, they experience a gradual process of 'social death' before they die in the physical sense. Those who are less dependent, however, are also confronted with this lack of interest.

Visiting older people is in most cases no longer an act with intrinsic social value – a 'pleasure'. Rather, it has become a moral duty one would rather not do. Ironically, it was only a foreign visitor who came to 'tap' their knowledge and wisdom. The growing loneliness of older and dependent people seems the clearest indication of their marginalisation and loss of social significance. The claim that older people are respected because of their wisdom and advanced age is a figure of speech, wishful and wistful thinking on the part of older people and only paid lip service by the younger generations. 'Respect' is first of all politeness; it is shown more by the deferential words of the young about older people than by their actual behaviour.

If loneliness is the 'unacceptable discrepancy between the amount and quality of actual social relationships compared with desired ones' (Perlman and Peplau, cited in Van Tilburg et al, 1998, 741) it is not difficult to determine which discrepancy is felt as the most painful by the older people in Kwahu-Tafo: the lack of interest of the younger generation in their wisdom and knowledge.

Ironically, loneliness can occur in spite of on-going social contacts; loneliness is most painful in the 'company' of people. Older people in Kwahu-Tafo, who are surrounded by the noise and bustle of everyday life and who seem the centre of respectful attention, are denied what they regard as their deepest existential right: the listening ear of a younger person.

Quality of care for older people

Care, both as a concept and as a practice, proved highly ambiguous.[3] The evasiveness of care as a research topic stems from the fact that people are likely to say very different things about the care they give or receive, depending on the context in which the conversation takes place and the mood of the person involved. Embarrassment over the little care they receive from their children may induce older people to conceal that painful truth and to praise their children for their love and good help. One does not wash one's dirty linen in the street, as the proverb goes in many languages including Twi: *Yensi yɛn ntamago wɔ abɔnten*. Yet the opposite may also occur. When an old person is in a bitter mood, he may be rather inclined to make his plight known and publicly accuse his relatives of negligence. The likelihood of such a reaction will increase further if the old person expects help from the one to whom he is talking.

The relatives and those who are supposed to provide care are also likely to produce contradictory accounts. They too may prefer to hide their shame of failing to provide proper care for the older people. They may otherwise opt to show openly their poverty and lack of means and their inability to provide care, hoping to get help from the listener. It is even possible to hear contradictory claims and complaints within one and the same interview. Finally, frustrations about the limited care given by fellow relatives may incite some to accuse their family members unduly of negligence.

The English term 'care' has various shades of meaning. Its two basic constituents are emotional and technical/practical. The latter refers to carrying out concrete activities for others who may not be able to do them by themselves. Parents take care of their children by feeding them, providing shelter, educating and training them, and so forth. Healthy people take care of sick ones and young people of old ones. Technically, care has a complementary character, one person completes another one. 'Care' also has an emotional meaning; it expresses concern, dedication and attachment. To do something with care or carefully implies that one acts with special devotion. The Twi term closest to 'care' is *hwɛ so* which literally means 'to look upon' or, more freely, 'to look after'.

Some of the most common activities for which older people need the help of others include: getting food, taking a bath, washing clothes and going to the toilet. Helping them financially and providing company are tokens of care, which are also indispensable. Finally and, in the eyes of many, the most important type of 'care' is the organisation of a fitting funeral when the older person dies.

Our observations and conversations in the town of Kwahu-Tafo resulted in an extremely diverse picture of care for older people. Some of them lived in blissful circumstances, others were outright miserable. I remember one older lady who was always surrounded by her three daughters who cared for her in a way one can only dream of. When we visited her she usually started to sing church hymns, praising both the Lord and her three daughters. The other extreme was an old man, lying on the floor of a bare room, blind and deserted by his children who lived only a few hundred metres from him but never came to visit him. When we came to him he begged us for money and tobacco and complained about his situation. A woman, distantly related, who happened to live in the same house, gave him the most basic things to stay alive. Between these two extremes we saw care in all different measures and kinds.

As mentioned before, whether older people actually get care in good quality and quantity depends on what they have achieved during their 'active' years. Those who have worked very hard and have taken good care of others, their children, their partners and other relatives, are most likely to receive care, attention and financial help. Getting good care in old age is foremost a matter of reciprocity. But, at the same time, reciprocity has only limited predictive power; people constantly deviate from the rules that they themselves formulate or they are unable to provide adequate care because of poverty.

There is not much reason for romanticising the situation of older people in Kwahu-Tafo. With the hazards of present-day life and the inability of many parents to give their children a safe foundation for a successful life, they may face considerable hardship in the last years of their lives. Minimal care will remain available to all older people, but a comfortable and pleasant old age will probably be reserved for a minority.

It is not unlikely that in a place like Kwahu-Tafo which is moving from a lineage-based community to a society of nuclear families and individuals, men will be the main victims of this 'calculating' provision of care. Where men, during their productive years, have shown to be little concerned about their children, they may expect the same lack of concern from their children in their old age. And where they have done little to support their wives they should reckon with the possibility that their wives will leave them.

Non-policy on welfare of older people

Welfare of older people is not perceived as a priority for Ghanaian politicians and policy makers. There is still a general assumption – or should we call it 'wishful thinking' – that Ghana is entirely different from 'western' societies in terms of kin solidarity. In Ghana, they emphasise that families look after their ageing members and will continue to do so. Handing over this responsibility to outsiders or professionals in institutions, as has become a common practice in many 'western' countries, is widely rejected in Ghana.

Politicians and opinion leaders are, however, not unaware of the fact that traditional family care is crumbling because of an economic, demographic and cultural transition. Government reports and articles in the popular press and on the Internet point out that Ghana is no more that 'youthful' country where older people are a small minority and are constantly surrounded by a host of younger relatives who both respect them and look after them.

Information from the Ghana Statistical Service shows that life expectancy at birth has increased to 60.7 years for men and 61.8 years for women and that life expectancy at the age of 60 has been estimated at 77.03 for men and 79.49 years for women. The 2010 Census results indicate that the population of people 60 years and above has increased to 6.7 per cent of the total population.[4]

The same sources also point out that family care for older people is going through a crisis. In fact, the alarm that is raised about this in government reports and popular media depicts conditions that are worse than I observed in my field research. I just emphasised the wide variety in quality of care, ranging from impressive examples of high quality family care to cases of extremely poor and lonely older people. But a government report is even more pessimistic:

- The majority of older people have not had the means or the opportunity to contribute to pension schemes that would assist in old age. Gratuity, pension schemes and related entitlements only cover the few older people who may have worked in the formal sector of the economy [and then primarily males, SvdG]. Small-scale farmers, fisher folks, craftsmen and petty traders do not benefit from these schemes.
- The benefits resulting from formal social security systems are in most cases inadequate and continuously lose purchasing power with inflation.
- Most people enter older age poor after a lifetime of poverty.
- Poor health and nutritional status inhibit older people's participation in income generating activities.
- Many older people are caring for those affected by HIV/AIDS which depletes any existing resources and limits their involvement in income generating opportunities.
- Poverty alleviation programmes tend to discriminate against older people.[5]

Manifestos of the major political parties going into elections in 2008 and 2012 announced the policy frameworks they had in mind for the older population of Ghana. The 'Livelihood Empowerment Against Poverty' (LEAP) programme was introduced by the NPP (New Patriotic Party) government in 2007, which the next government found prudent to continue. LEAP is described as 'the flagship programme of Ghana's National Social Protection Strategy that aims to create an all-inclusive and socially-empowered society through the provision of sustainable mechanisms for the protection of people living in extreme poverty, related vulnerability and exclusion'. The focus is on children, disabled people, those who are chronically sick and people with HIV/AIDS. Older people are also listed as beneficiaries but seem to benefit little from the programme.[6] Older people *are*, however, entitled to free health care under the present National Health Insurance Scheme (NHIS). To what extent that entitlement is indeed realised is not clear. A few years ago the Vice President of HelpAge Ghana stated that the NHIS disregards the special geriatric health needs of older people: 'The NHIS prescribes the same basic health care without taking into consideration the tertiary health care needs of older people especially in the area of non-communicable diseases such as retention of urine, incontinence, prostrate and colon cancers.'[7]

The most elaborate government report on its (intended) policy toward the improvement of welfare for older people, 'National ageing policy: Ageing with security and dignity' (Government of Ghana, 2010), lists all the key words and rhetoric provided by the Second World Assembly on Ageing in Madrid (2002), focusing on the alleviation of poverty and increasing the independency of older people. Most relevant, however, is the suggestions of the report for older people who are no longer able to work and fully depend on the care of the family. Particularly urgent is the question to what extent the old principle of economic and social reciprocity as a basis for adequate care is still viable today. Will the family be able to continue its traditional care in a time where demographic and economic changes, and in its wake, drifting family values, lead to a very different society?

Aboderin (2006), having studied intergenerational support and care for older people in an urban context, reached similar conclusions to what I found in the rural context of Kwahu. She pointed out that filial obligations to the older generation are changing and middle-aged parents are gradually shifting their priorities from their ageing parents to their own children. She pleads for a 'right balance of family and state responsibility for securing the welfare of the growing older population, and ways in which family support systems can be strengthened' (p 164).

Introducing a fair pension system that also covers the approximate 75 per cent of older people who never worked in formal employment (and – therefore – have not directly contributed to a pension) seems, however, a far cry in the 2010 government report.[8] There is no indication that the government seriously considers such a step. The following text excels in vagueness:

> 4.7.3 Government will vigorously pursue the implementation of the revised and new three-tier pension scheme including the establishment of systems and processes for capturing Ghanaians working in the informal economy into the scheme.

The report also does not contemplate providing institutional care for older people who have no means and no people to support them, those who are financially and – what is more important – socially indigent. The term 'care institute' – or a synonym – is not even mentioned as an option in the 2010 report.

The only 'concrete' suggestion in the report to improve the welfare of the most vulnerable older people is harking back to the values of the past when families are believed really to have cared for their older members. Assuming for a moment that that interpretation of the past is correct, one wonders if the authors of the report do not realise that values of the past cannot be simply transferred to another time with a very different economic and demographic structure. The following quote shows the 'philosophy' that policy makers seem to adhere to when they ponder the improvement of livelihood conditions of the older generation.

> 4.6.2 Government will promote interventions that strengthen solidarity between generations especially in families and communities to ensure that Ghana is a society for all generations. Family and community solidarity will be strengthened and intergenerational ties at the family and community levels will be vigorously promoted. Public education on ageing including the promotion of positive images of older people will be promoted to broaden the understanding of ageing, avoid generational segregation, strengthening solidarity among generations, promote mutual, productive exchange between generations and also achieve reciprocity between generations at the family and community levels.

> 4.6.3 Efforts will be made to uphold the traditional family structures and norms such that it will be able to provide the needed support for older relatives. The family will be encouraged to develop plans and incorporate in these plans strategies to support older people in the family. The family will be assisted to identify, support and strengthen traditional support systems to enhance the abilities of families and communities to care for older family members.

The authors of the report *are* aware that conditions have changed for families:

6.2.1 Presently, family structures are changing and traditional patterns of care are no longer guaranteed. Migration of the economically active population from rural areas to urban centres has resulted in many older people living alone in rural areas. Difficult economic situations and changing social values have made families either unable or unwilling to care for older relatives.

The same authors seem to forget this observation the next moment, however, when they jump again to unfounded moralistic exhortations:

6.2.2 The family will continue to remain the most important source of support of older people. The social welfare and social protection structures will increase focus, attention and resources for the family. Government will ensure that traditional values and norms inform national and district level policies with regard to family values and the care of older people.

How is such a spectacular reversal possible?

6.2.3...Government will implement policies and programmes aimed at ensuring that the family and community change their attitude towards older relatives. The family and community will also be supported to avail themselves with education and training programmes targeted at improving caregiving to older people. The family particularly will be made to seek continuous capacity enhancement to enable it to care adequately for older family members. Families and communities will further be required to liaise with the social welfare as well as at the district level and also establish durable partnership arrangements with key stakeholders who provide support to older people.

The lack of vision is startling and the failure to see developments in their historical context naïve. The authors seem unaware of the social and moral complexities that led to the present crisis. Interestingly, they call for research to inform policy on the ageing population:

6.1.12 Universities and research institutions have a key role to play in shaping policy on older people. The *paucity of data* [emphasis added, SvdG] has been identified as one of the major constraining factors for inadequate planning and programming for older people in Ghana.

A generous concession, but they seem unaware of the research that *has* been done. Occasionally there is a reference to (mostly vague) statistical data, but more qualitative research that analyses the emic views and experiences of family members and older people regarding care and wellbeing of older people is totally ignored. The work by Apt (1993; 1996; 2002), Aboderin (2004; 2006), Van der Geest (1997; 2002; 2004), Darkwa (2000) and Dsane (2010), for example, seems unknown or is ignored by those who are supposed to design a policy for a better future for older people. The gap between research and policy rather than the paucity of research is the problem. There is no uptake of the valuable existing research. The reasons behind this wasteful oversight remain unclear. Have the writers of the report failed to do their homework or have they ignored the existing literature on purpose? Did they find it irrelevant or its implications too cumbersome, or too expensive?

Local initiatives and resistance

In the meantime, families, social and religious organisations and private entrepreneurs seek their own solutions to the crisis of care for older people, knowing that little can be expected from a government that does not even seem to know – or chooses to ignore – what takes place on the ground.

Families try creative ways to overcome their dilemmas. Matching grandchildren and grandparents, as is described by Douglas Frimpong-Nnuroh (no date) in his research among older people in Nzema society, is one such experiment. Relatives who have migrated to higher-income societies try to compensate their absence at home by sending money to their aged parents or relatives to enable them to provide or 'buy' decent care. Cati Coe (2014, 161) in her book on the 'scattered' Ghanaian family (referring to transnational families) also points at the 'repertoire' of reciprocal care that migrated parents organise by leaving their children with their grandmothers. A number of families (no statistics are available) have such absentee relatives who make 'distant-care' possible through remittances.

Families that can afford it (often thanks to foreign remittances) are now increasingly 'employing' more distant relatives or non-relatives to provide care in the home of the older people.[9] Sometimes they also hire medical personnel, often a nurse, who comes every so often, in addition to the live-in caregiver.

Organisations such as churches and NGOs experiment with daycare centres in urban areas. During 2006, I visited such a centre that was run by a Catholic organisation in Accra. The older people who attended the centre played games or did simple handicrafts and were given a generous lunch. Nowadays, more such centres exist, some also run by private entrepreneurs, but a reliable overview of the number and quality of such centres does not exist. A message from HelpAge Ghana in 2011 suggests that such centres may be facing several problems:

> The ageing population in the country is likely to be bored stiff as the only and first-ever ageing support centre in the country – HelpAge Ghana has been temporarily closed down due to over population [due to an overwhelming demand for its services].[10] The non-governmental, non-religious and non-profit making organization which has been operational since 1988 served as a recreational health care centre for retirees and other seniors who did not have anything or anyone to occupy their time with...In an interview with *The Globe* newspaper, Vice President of HelpAge Ghana, Edward Ameyibor, said the activities of the organization would have been more effective if they had more philanthropic support...'We used to provide three square meals each day at the centres, but it got to a time they started complaining about the quality of food. Then we started preparing different kinds of meals but at the cost of 50 pesewas each day but that also didn't work out...we closed down the centre, not just because of the food but also because our facility didn't have the capacity to handle the rising numbers of members.'[11, 12]

The statement of the vice president echoes the comments in the introduction of this chapter about imagined old people's homes in Ghana: too expensive and too popular to be viable. The crux is that the price of creating residential infrastructure is prohibitive. Returning to the possibility of centres that provide 24-hour care to older people: the persistent silence about this option in policy documents and the outspoken rejection of this 'western' phenomenon by moral leaders suggest that institutional care for older people will not be a realistic and culturally acceptable solution for Ghana's present crisis, as is the contention in most Sub-Saharan African countries.

A Catholic bishop (Sarpong, 1983), for example, is quoted, 'We must desist from creating…such dead ends into Ghanaian life. For me, the day we adopt such a culturally humiliating system will be a gloomy one indeed. Let us continue to keep the aged in their homes with their children and grandchildren.' More recently, a Ghanaian blogger Dr Kwame Osei decries the decadent impact of 'the West' on Ghana. His long list of complaints includes the western treatment of older people:

> In the West it is quite commonplace for young people to disrespect their elders and for them to be placed in old people's homes when they become old. In Ghana this disregard for our elderly is not AFRIKAN and is something that we MUST rectify if we as a people are to regain our dignity, principles and moral values. (Osei, 2010)[13]

At the same time, however, the earlier mentioned trend to hire non-relatives for home-based care of older people seems a development in the direction of formal professional care. Sarah Dsane (2013) described the ambivalence of Ga families towards care of older people by 'strangers'; on the one hand they reject this option in strong terms but on the other hand two initiatives in Accra of care by outsiders do seem to attract some older people of families that are unable to provide the quality of care that their older relatives need and deserve. One of those initiatives is a residential home; the other is a home-care service by professional caregivers.

The Mercy Home Care Centre in Accra is an initiative of a Ghanaian couple living in Switzerland. They emphasise that the centre is not a commercial enterprise and that the payments made by families (370 Ghana Cedi per month, about £63) do not cover the costs of residence. The home started somewhere in 2012. When I visited the centre with Sarah Dsane in October 2013, there were nine residents whereas there was room for 30. One condition for acceptance is that families visit their older relative at least once a week. The four staff members (at the level of clinical health assistant or below) live in the building and are permanently available, seven days a week, day and night. When we talk to some of the residents, they admit that they did not feel happy at first, but now they show understanding for the decision of their children who were too busy to take proper care of them. Some residents only stay for a short period while their caregiver at home is not available. The centre is neat and simple and not meant for affluent people who will find it easy to hire professional help staying with them in their own home. It is unclear if this initiative will be sustainable.

The other initiative is Ripples Health Care (an NGO established in 2003), which is not a nursing home, but provides palliative care to terminally ill individuals in their own homes. It also offers care for the mentally and physically challenged. Although the older people are not mentioned as possible clients, they are included. I was not able to visit their office but the NGO has an elaborate and informative website. It also has its own training programme for caregivers. Both initiatives could be pioneering experiments with non-family caregiving to older people.

It may be useful to point out that the tradition of keeping older people within the family is not typically Ghanaian or African; it used to be a global tradition. Less than a hundred years ago in the Netherlands (my home country), many older people lived with or near their children and grandchildren and performed all kinds of activities in and around the house. It would be a mistake to say that old people's homes belong to the 'western' tradition; they are a recent phenomenon. Most of these institutions in the Netherlands were only established about 75 years ago.[14] It would also be a mistake to assume that Dutch people wholeheartedly choose for the option of institutional care. In most cases the decision is taken with regret and pain but regarded as the least harmful of several difficult options.

One can only speculate over the question whether the changes which took place in 'western' societies will also occur in Ghana. I believe that they will eventually, in spite of the rhetoric to the opposite. The increased importance of paid employment, the growing mobility, the widening generation gap, the demographic changes and even the economic growth, which led to care institutions and formal care programmes in the Netherlands, can already be witnessed in Ghana.

Will, alternatively, Ghanaian families, NGOs, churches or 'social entrepreneurs' – I do not expect much initiative from the government – be able to come up with other options? In South Africa NGOs experiment with the model of assisted living communities, where NGOs acquire small neighbouring houses that each accommodate six to ten older people, who are able to lead a 'normal' (home-like) existence (co-residence), and benefit from care/help from co-residents (Ferreira, 2013). They are not alone or lonely and have a parent organisation to keep an eye on their welfare. There seems to be no stigma attached to such residences.[15] Scant descriptions of various forms of institutionalised care for older people are also reported from other African countries, such as Zambia (Sichingabula, 2000a; 2000b; Report, 2011[16]), Zimbabwe (Nyanguru, 1987; Mupedziswa, 1998), and DR Congo (Pype, Chapter Two).

Conclusion

My question was whether Ghanaian families would be able to continue providing day-to-day care to their ageing grandparents when they become dependent, or will economic growth and improvement of medical care with the ensuing lengthening of life eventually lead to 'the development of formal care programmes' in Ghana? In the not too distant future, Ghanaians will become even more mobile, will have fewer children, will live increasingly in nuclear families and will grow older. In that same future families will find it more and more difficult to provide good care for their ageing relatives and will look for new alternatives of care.

The Ghana government seems to turn a blind eye to the economic, demographic and 'cultural' developments that have led to the present crisis in family care for older people. It is relying on rhetoric that allows it to ignore the responsibility it has towards its older and frail citizens. The report cited earlier reduces the crisis of care for older people to a moral problem that should be solved by re-educating families and seems unwilling to learn from the experiences in 'western' societies that went through a similar transition less than a century ago. Unwillingness and inability to provide tangible and effective support to its ageing citizens is camouflaged with calls for a revival of traditional values. As mentioned before, the government's policy presents a stark contradiction to its own diagnosis of the problems that caregivers face but it also has political logic: by blaming families for neglecting their older relatives and calling for a return to the virtues of the past it tries to keep up the appearance of good governance.

Dsane's (2013) exploration of professional non-kin-based care for frail older people in Ghana seems to suggest that middle-class and well-to-do families may find their own solution for this challenge. Initiatives to relieve the burden of care for the majority of poor families are, however, practically unknown.

I am not suggesting that Ghana – and for that matter other African societies – should rush out to adopt the 'western' model of institutional care of older people. It seems even ludicrous to hold up the most advanced long-term care housing models in the world for the Ghanaian government to emulate. The aim of this chapter was rather to highlight the unrealistic attitude of Ghanaian policy-makers and their – calculated(?) – lack of foresight. Experiences of countries that were confronted and had to deal with the consequences of demographic transition should be studied in earnest to develop a suitable and just policy for older people in Ghana.

Notes

[1] Interestingly, Emily Freeman (Chapter Five) writing about rural Malawi, emphasises that older people's dependency on their children (which in Ghana is a sign of a successful life) is frowned upon: 'Inability to care for oneself was universally referenced as a bad old age.' Self-reliance is an indication of success in old age.

[2] This section draws on Van der Geest (2004).

[3] This section draws on Van der Geest (2002).

[4] www.ghanabusinessnews.com/2012/10/02/ghana-govt-to-present-bill-on-national-ageing-policy-to-parliament/

[5] Government of Ghana (2010) National Ageing Policy of Ghana: Ageing with security and dignity, www.ghanaweb.com/GhanaHomePage/blogs/blog.article.php?blog=3442&ID=1000008901

[6] Personal communication, Douglas Frimpong-Nnuroh, on the basis of his research in the Nzema area.

[7] www.ghanabusinessnews.com/2013/04/19/nhis-neglecting-health-needs-of-older-people-helpage-ghana/

[8] Pensions for all older people are rare in Africa; they exist – in different forms and degrees – only in South Africa, Botswana, Lesotho, Mauritius, Swaziland and Namibia (Scodellaro, 2010) as well as Zanzibar.

[9] This trend is common in southern European countries where live-in migrant caregivers are hired by the family to look after their ageing parents (see Van der Geest et al, 2002). Hiring a private caregiver is regarded a better (less visible and therefore less shameful) option than sending the parent to a care institution.

[10] HelpAge Ghana was not the 'only and first-ever ageing support centre in the country'; several religious organisations had been experimenting with daycare activities at local levels.

[11] www.citifmonline.com/index.php

[12] In a comment Monica Ferreira, social gerontologist from South Africa, added: 'The senior centre (or luncheon club) movement is very big in South Africa. Senior centres are run by NGOs and subsidised by the government based on membership. Typically, members arrive at about 10 am, have tea and eat, engage in activities, such as

handicrafts, or may listen to talks or play games. Men and women have separate pursuits; culturally, there is no mingling. Health education may be offered, or training in human rights. There may be counselling offered. Some centres offer basic health care and are even approved to dispense prescribed chronic medications. *The highlight is a cooked lunch* [emphasis added]...Apart from the pension, the centres are the government's main welfare programme for older people. Senior centres are the mainstay of formal welfare support to older people in South Africa.' In his contribution to this volume, Jaco Hoffman (Chapter Seven) points out that South Africa's old age pension is an important obstacle to institutional care for older people, since families fear losing the older person's pension when he/she moves out of the house to an institution.

[13] The literature about institutional care in so-called developing or low-income countries is confusing and contradictory. In Kinshasa, Democratic Republic of Congo, inhabitants of retirement homes feel excluded from society but now seem to obtain 'a new kind of value' and 'social function', according to Katrien Pype (Chapter Two). In India, it is reported that old people's homes are becoming more common and acceptable for well-to-do older people as well as for older people who have no relatives with whom to stay (Mishra, 2004; Hahn, 2005). An Indian woman responded, however, that it is still seen as a failure on the part of children to fulfil their responsibility: 'There is not a single example around me in my extended family or social network where the elders are living in an old age home...My Mom uses it to emotionally blackmail me...that maybe she should just go and live in an old age home...(telling me, I don't care enough for her)' (personal communication from Indian anthropologist).

[14] There were some charity homes for destitute older people in the cities from around the sixteenth century onwards. They had, however, a very different character to the present old people's homes.

[15] Personal communication, Monica Ferreira.

[16] The Report (2011, 13) observed that the conditions in the nine homes for care of older people in Zambia 'were deplorable, under financed and in most instances overcrowded. In addition, these old age homes were very limited in number and could not cater for all the old people that needed care.'

Acknowledgements
I thank Patrick Atuobi, Yaw Obeng Boamah, Benjamin Boadu, Jaco Hoffman, Katrien Pype, Cati Coe, Josien de Klerk and Douglas Frimpong-Nnuroh for their various ways of helping me with this chapter. I am particularly grateful to Monica Ferreira who provided extensive critical comments on an earlier version.

References

Aboderin, I, 2004, Decline in material family support for older people in urban Ghana, Africa: Understanding processes and causes of change, *Journal of Gerontology: Psychological Sciences, Social Sciences* 59, S128–S137

Aboderin, I, 2006, *Intergenerational support and old age in Africa*, London: Transaction Publishers

Apt, NA, 1993, Care of the elderly in Ghana: An emerging issue, *Journal of Cross-Cultural Gerontology* 8, 1, 301–12

Apt, NA, 1996, *Coping with old age in a changing Africa: Social change and the elderly Ghanaian*, Aldershot: Avebury

Apt, NA, 2002, Ageing and the changing role of the family and the community: An African perspective, *International Social Security Review* 55, 39–47

Atobrah, D, 2009, Caring for the chronically sick within Ga families: A study of modern innovations and traditional practices, Unpublished dissertation, University of Ghana

Atobrah, D, 2013, Behold! The sweet and sour soup: Globalization and family care for cancer patients in Ghana, Paper presented at the international conference 'Revisiting the first international congress of Africanists in a globalised world', 24–26 October, Institute of African Studies, University of Ghana

Coe, C, 2014, *The scattered family: Parenting, African migrants and global inequality*, Chicago, IL: University of Chicago Press

Darkwa, OK, 2000, Toward a comprehensive understanding of the needs of elderly Ghanaians, *Ageing International* 25, 4, 65–79

Dsane, S, 2010, Care of the elderly: A case study of grandmothers and childless elderly women in Teshie, PhD thesis, Legon: University of Ghana

Dsane, S, 2013, Can 'strangers' provide care for frail older people in Ga families?, Paper, presented at the international conference 'Revisiting the first international congress of Africanists in a globalised world', 24–26 October, Institute of African Studies, University of Ghana

Ferreira, M, 2013, South Africa, www.ilc-alliance.org/images/uploads/publication-pdfs/ILC-South_Africa.pdf

Freeman, E, 2016, Care and identity in rural Malawi, this volume

Frimpong-Nnuroh, D, no date, Intergenerational relations and care in an era of globalization: A study of grandparents and grandchildren in Ellembelle Nzema, Ghana, Draft PhD thesis, University of Amsterdam, in progress

Government of Ghana, 2010, National ageing policy: Ageing with security and dignity, Accra: Government of Ghana, Ministry of Employment and Social Welfare

Hahn, B, 2005, Happy endings: An ethnographic account of elderly women's life at the House of Providence. Unpublished master thesis, Medical Anthropology, University of Amsterdam

Hoffman, J, 2016, Negotiating care for older persons in South Africa: Between the ideal and the pragmatics, this volume

ILC (International Longevity Centre), 2013, Housing for older people globally: What are the best practices? An ILC Global Alliance Discussion Paper, www.ilc-alliance.org/index.php/home

Mishra, AJ, 2004, The elderly in India: A study of old age home residents in Orissa. Unpublished doctoral dissertation, Indian Institute of Technology Kanpur

Mupedziswa, R, 1998, Community living for destitute older Zimbabweans: Institutional care with a human face, *Southern African Journal of Gerontology* 7, 1, 26–31

Nyanguru, AC, 1987, Residential care for the destitute elderly: A comparative study of two institutions in Zimbabwe, *Journal of Cross-Cultural Gerontology* 2, 345–57

Osei, K, 2010, Western culture: The cause of Ghana's decadent society, www.modernghana.com/news/297270/1/western-culture-the-cause-of-ghanas-decadent-socie.html

Pype, K, 2016, Caring for people with and without value: Movement, reciprocity and respect in Kinshasa's retirement homes, this volume

Report, 2011, Report of the Committee on Health, Community Development and Social Welfare for the first session of the eleventh National Assembly, Lusaka: National Assembly of Zambia

Sarpong, PK, 1983, Ageing and tradition, in J Opare-Abetia (ed) *Ageing and social change: A Ghanaian perspective*, pp 13–20, Legon: Institute of Adult Education

Scodellaro, C, 2010, Les articulations entre solidarités publiques et solidarités privées en Afrique du Sud: les pensions vieillesse et leurs effets, *Autrepart* 53, 57–74.

Sichingabula, YM, 2000a, The provision of housing and care for older persons in Lusaka, Zambia, *Southern African Journal of Gerontology* 9, 1, 10–14

Sichingabula, YM, 2000b, An environmental assessment of Divine Providence Home in Lusaka, Zambia, *Southern African Journal of Gerontology* 9, 1, 25–9

Van der Geest, S, 1997, Money and respect: The changing value of old age in rural Ghana, *Africa* 67, 4, 534–59

Van der Geest, S, 2002, Respect and reciprocity: Care of elderly people in rural Ghana', *Journal of Cross-Cultural Gerontology* 17, 1, 3–31

Van der Geest, S, 2004, 'They don't come to listen': The experience of loneliness among older people in Kwahu, Ghana, *Journal of Cross-Cultural Gerontology* 19, 2, 77–96

Van der Geest, S, Mul, A, Vermeulen, H, 2002, Linkages between migration and care for older people: Observations from Greece, Ghana and the Netherlands, *Ageing and Society* 24, 431–50

Van Tilburg, TH, De Jong Gierveld, J, Lechini, L, Marsiglia, D, 1998, Social integration and loneliness: A comparative study among older adults in the Netherlands and Tuscany, Italy, *Journal of Social and Personal Relationships* 15, 6, 740–54

Caring for people 'without' value: movement, reciprocity and respect in Kinshasa's retirement homes

Katrien Pype

Introduction

Currently, Kinshasa counts eight retirement homes (Fr. Sg. *home de vieillards*, *hospice*),[1] the oldest of which dates from 1943. Five of these homes were built during colonial times (the Democratic Republic of Congo gained its independence in 1960), while three others were added over the years: one (in the neighbourhood of Kingabwa, and attached to the parish of St Kizito, with which it shares its name) was built during the early 1970s by the Congolese Catholic Church; another one, also in the early 1970s, was constructed by the Catholic association Soeurs des Pauvres de Bergamo (Kingasani), and the most recent *hospice*, financed with Catholic money, was started by a Congolese woman (Kingabwa). These homes differ significantly in capacity: most can accommodate 30 residents, while two could easily house 80 residents. However, none of these retirement homes is fully operational. During fieldwork (2011–13), there were about 120 *indigents* (the common appellation for retirement home residents) living in these homes. In a city of more than eight million inhabitants, this is a very small number. Generally, these spaces have not been the focus of academic study; nor are many Kinois (inhabitants of Kinshasa) familiar with the retirement homes. Nevertheless, there is a constant flow of movement between city and retirement homes, and vice versa (see Photo 2.2). The city's possibly best-known *hospice* (on Avenue Cabinda, opposite the national broadcasting services) has turned into a recreational space where journalists and local celebrities drink and eat in *malewa* (small outdoor restaurants) developed on the retirement home's premises. The land on which the home is located is also constantly invaded by soccer-playing youth. The children drink from the water pump and refresh themselves under the gaze of older

Photo 2.1: Dolls made by an indigent and sold by her on the pavement in front of the retirement home next to small, non-perishable items such as batteries, matches and pens (© Katrien Pype, 2013)

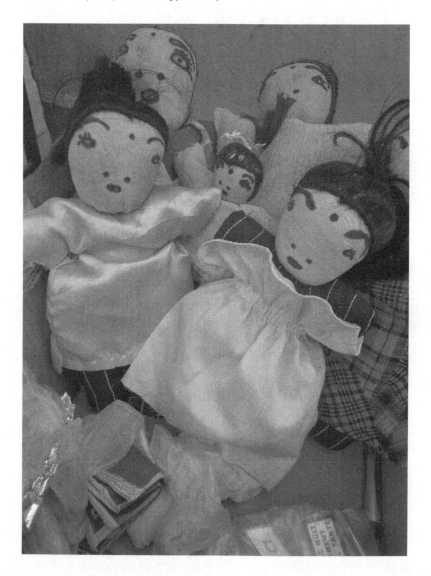

people, while neighbours fetch water for household use. The residents of this and other *hospices* send children on errands, or sell cigarettes and personally made goods to visitors and passers-by (see Photo 2.1). In addition, after work hours (usually after 5 pm), *indigents* venture out of the retirement home and start begging on the street. These are only a few examples of the constant interaction between older residents and the city at large.

This chapter aims to bring the retirement home into the conversation about care services in African societies. While there are indeed not that many retirement homes operating on the continent, they nonetheless exist and are part of the urban landscape. The *homes de vieillards* constitute one category among the various spaces of care[2] available in the city. Hospitals, rehabilitation centres, compounds of tradi-practitioners and *nganga* (healers and diviners), orphanages, but also places such as churches (see Hoffman, Chapter Seven), family houses (see Obrist, Chapter Four and Van Eeuwijk, Chapter Three), associations for older people and informal support groups where care is provided in less formal ways, can all be called 'spaces of care'. By focusing on how retirement homes are situated within these various spaces of care and the overall urban environment, and by focusing in particular on how movement in and out of these spaces occurs – that is, for example, why are elderly people in retirement homes? – this chapter addresses larger themes such as intergenerational relations in contemporary Africa, urban infrastructure and public services. An ethnography of urban space, care and older people will unsettle the image of the African city as a space of youth, will hopefully provide a new grid for 'the urban experience', and will contribute to the anthropology of old age/ageing (Keith, 1980; Myerhoff, 1978; Sokolovsky, 1997; Spencer, 1990; Aguilar, 1998; Lamb, 2000; Makoni and Stroeken, 2002), which has long focused on health problems and intergenerational relations (Hurwicz, 1995; Hareven, 1996; Obrist et al, 2003; Alber et al, 2004; Van Eeuwijk and Obrist, 2006; Van der Geest and Whyte, 2008). While for obvious reasons youth have been a privileged category in anthropological analyses of post-colonial African urban lifeworlds (Honwana and De Boeck, 2005; Christiansen et al, 2006; Cole and Durham, 2008), an approach to the city's 'spaces of care', and in particular an analysis of the social spaces where senior residents are being cared for, brings novel perspectives on urban livelihoods.

Material for this chapter was collected through participant fieldwork in the context of a larger study on the lifeworlds of Kinshasa's elderly residents,[3] with a special focus on their experience of the mediatised urban environment. Between 2011 and 2013, I have conducted 12 months of fieldwork on the topic: visiting elderly people in their homes, accompanying them to the hospital, to church, to visit relatives and to their associations. Three months were almost entirely devoted to visiting retirement homes where, together with Marie-Jeanne

Musito, a researcher in an anthropology research group (CERDAS) at the University of Kinshasa, I conducted a series of interviews with retirement home residents and staff.

The first part of this chapter examines perceptions about older people in the city, followed by an exploration of retirement homes, with a particular focus on how Kinois talk about these spaces, and how older people manipulate common opinions about them. Thereafter the chapter investigates retirement homes as spaces of movement. By describing how elderly people arrive in retirement homes and how the city constantly moves in and out of these *hospices*, this chapter attempts to make the retirement home visible in the study of African societies. I use pseudonyms when giving voice to research participants for privacy reasons.

Being 'old' in Kinshasa

In a country like Democratic Republic of Congo, where life expectancy does not reach beyond the age of 48, anyone who has passed this landmark by a few years or more is regarded as 'an elderly person' (*vieux*). Yet, an 'elderly person' is someone who has gone through various social and physical processes in his or her life. Different concepts are used to indicate these processes. The Lingala word *mukolo* refers to an adult, mature person (as opposed to *mwana*, a child). *Kokola* – the verb from which *mukolo* is derived – means first and foremost 'to grow up', but mainly denotes people who have taken on social responsibilities (in particular having dependents like a wife and [classificatory] children around him). *Mubange*, on the other hand, indicates a physically old person, often with a 'tired' body. *Bakoko* could be translated as 'grandparents', and situates older people within a social world, usually the family, but it could also be used more anonymously: the elders in the city. The French *vieux* is used both in the relative and in the absolute meanings. Much like 'youth' (Durham, 2000), the notion of 'an old person' (*un vieux*) is a social shifter, that is, apart from having an absolute sense of the concept of 'an elder' (*mobange, moto akoli* 'someone who has grown', *mukolo, koko*) in contemporary Kinshasa, being 'old' is a relative (relational) identity. Respect and authority are given to people who are older than you: one shows respect to one's seniors and is oneself also a senior to one's juniors, who in turn need to show respect to you.

Other, politico-economic understandings of 'being old' also exist in Kinois society. People working for private companies or the government can retire at the age of 65.[4] While 65 might be a modern, political-economic invention fixing the boundaries between those who are still industrious, that is physically capable to labour in/for society, and those whose bodies are becoming tired and thus who are no longer 'useful' in society, for most Kinois, as soon as people have reached their mid-50s or early 60s, they are 'old'.

Elderly people are both socially and physically a minority in Kinshasa. This city with more than eight million inhabitants is just like any other African city: a space where youth dominate. In popular culture, in the streets, and even in the (formal and informal) economies, the youth are said to be setting the tune. Unsurprisingly then, old people are the objects of jokes: it is said that they do not know how to behave in the city; they do not know how to dress well, how to speak French; they are not up to date on the newest technologies. Also, they are often blamed for the hardships their children and grandchildren are experiencing. Furthermore, the life stage 'youth' has come to be considered more powerful because of the privileges young people enjoy on the formal economic market. Young men and women not only outnumber older people in society at large, they are also socially and economically very influential: job offers with foreign NGOs or companies are primarily addressed to students, who then fill the vacant positions, have incomes, and bring money home. Other important money-generating activities in which young people generally engage – like petty commerce or brokering economic transactions (among them prostitution, fraud and extortion) – are more lucrative than whatever efforts their parents or older relatives make.[5] In such contexts, gerontocracy cannot be upheld for long (also Aguilar, 1998).

The social esteem for 'youth' is so prominent that even the social identity of a '*jeune*' has become more desirable than that of '*vieux*', typically regarded as the most respected social identity in Africa, or as the main expression of authority and respect. Discourse about the musician Papa Wemba illustrates how the familiar boundaries between young and old have been overhauled. Because of his age (in June 2012, he celebrated his 63rd birthday),[6] Papa Wemba should be talked about as an 'old person' (*mukolo* – someone who has aged). Yet, because this musician sustains Kinshasa's nightlife with sensual performances, continues to enrich the vocabulary of seduction and courtship, dresses very elegantly and refuses to take on the bodily habitus of an elder (immobile, silent and stern looking), but instead behaves in a youthful and playful manner, many Kinois talk about him as a *false youth* (*un faux jeune*), that is: an old man behaving like a young person. Others talk about him as *jeune premier* – something like 'first class youth'. Many men in their 40s, 50s, and even in their early 60s take Papa Wemba as a role model and prefer to be called '*jeune*' as well. Thus both the urban economy and the music world have contributed to the decrease of seniority's appeal.

This urban idiom of 'youth' affects social relations between younger and older people, and also transforms the quality of the social prestige bestowed on the category of 'the elderly person'.[7] Societal ideals prescribe that elderly people should be met with respect, fear, deference and silence. Romantic ideas of older people as having been able to accumulate more wisdom than the younger generations, as well as more mystical interpretations whereby they possess harmful occult powers, are often invoked when explaining why one should fear, obey and not contradict an elderly person. In practice, however, not all elders in Kinshasa are constantly met with these honours. Rather, seniors who are suspected of being *bandoki* (Lingala Sg. *ndoki*, a person with mystical powers), sick elders whose caregiving has become a burden for their offspring, or quarrelsome elders, are abused, mocked and socially isolated or even abandoned. Especially, according to young Pentecostals, the 'paganism' of older people, that is, their knowledge of tradition and assumed participation in customary practices (in a Pentecostal language understood as demonic behaviour, and thus sinful), is the reason for the hardships the young are experiencing. Significant in this Pentecostal context is the fact that the youths equate their elders with *féticheurs*: older people are perceived as being no different than experts of the invisible. A recurring expression among Kinshasa's young people runs: 'The word of an elder person is like the word of a *féticheur*' (*Lilobi bakulutu, bilobi banganga*). This refers to the magical power of older people's speech: what they say can become reality, just as a diviner can produce the future through his words. I will return to this issue of *kindoki* (the capacity of mystically intervening in reality, thus combining witchcraft and sorcery, whether for the good or the bad) below. 'In many Congolese ethnic groups, it is dangerous to grow old,' as the late Professor Tshungu, a Congolese colleague, told me during one of our conversations.

Older people also reflect on their position in society, and many regret having become *moto pamba*, literally, people lacking everything. While the concept *moto pamba* is mainly used to indicate 'poor people', and while for many elderly deprivation is a reality, there are also more symbolic usages of the term, mainly referring to people without any value. Here, having value is a relational concept, because it is others who recognise value in a person. In a general sense, *bato pamba* are people who do not contribute to society, older people who designate themselves as *bato pamba* always immediately refer to their families, for whom they have become 'worthless people' (see Van der Geest, Chapter One).

Money, however, seems to provide a protective shield against physical and social abandonment. Van der Geest (1997, 536) describes how, in rural Ghana, elderly residents with money are respected. He argues that older people who made money in the past and have been able to give their children a 'good' life, 'should not be worried about their old days, since [care] will be given by their children and other relatives who have benefited from their hard work' (1997, 555). The same goes for Kinshasa's society, where older people who are physically capable of working usually remain economically active as long as possible.[8] Yet, since the start of the economic crisis in the early 1980s, an increasing number of older people have never been able to give their offspring a 'good life'. It is often argued that older people who receive a pension from the state have the best guarantees for being well-treated by their offspring, who are themselves in dire need of that (often very minimal) pension to feed, shelter and educate children and grandchildren.

As a result, gerontocracy has suffered a lot from the privileges 'youth' gained in the economy, and elders are regarded as ambivalent figures. The ways in which Kinois approach older people vary and cover a whole gamut of emotions (ranging from pride and deepest respect to aversion and fear). Older people are at once feared for being *bandoki*, respected for being life-givers, rejected for being burdensome, and approached for being knowledgeable because of their life experience; they are objects of mockery and of esteem; they are to be consulted and to be asked for advice; they are simultaneously parents and children (because they need to be nurtured like small children).[9]

These approaches towards older people (self-designations as well as more collective understandings of the position of seniors in society), however, obscure the various spaces in which older people do remain active and find meaning and self-worth. Examples are the various folkloric music and dance bands, where elderly men take leading roles as choreographers, singers and musicians. These groups perform during funerals, ethnic-related meetings and at neighbourhood-oriented parties. Also, older people are members of ethnic-based, region-based and religious or professional associations, where, as long as they are mobile, they meet, support[10] and entertain one another. In addition, a small section of Kinshasa's popular culture is directed towards older people, and stages the 'urban elderly', that is those who were young and residing in the city during the 1950s and 1960s, as experts of the urban music scene (music TV shows such as *Bana Leo*, *Sentiment Lipopo* (Pype, 2017)).

Houses of *bandoki*

In Kinshasa, the ideal relationship towards one's elders is contained within the French verb *s'occuper de* or the slang *kokipe na*, literally, 'to take care of' or 'to see to'. This verb contains various meanings: it means to feed, to clothe, to house ageing parents, ensure their health, and also make sure that older people feel respected and loved. The French verb *soigner* is also often used when talking about how to live with one's elderly relatives. *Soigner* means 'taking special care of', being careful with them, with their bodies and minds, because they are vulnerable, and perceived as individuals at risk. As mentioned above, older people are also perceived as risky individuals themselves. Very much like children and young people, elderly people are perceived with a great deal of ambiguity (see Honwana and De Boeck, 2005). In particular, as one grows older, one is also more vulnerable to accusations of possessing supernatural powers that can be used either for good or evil (*kindoki*). Therefore, it is important not to vex your seniors, even those living in the village, people told me, and new-born children need to have the blessing of their grandparents for a healthy and successful life. Moreover, on a larger collective level, the accumulation of mystical powers in the bodies of the aged is acknowledged. It is illustrative that the national football team requested that the residents of the retirement home in [Avenue] Cabinda pray during one of their recent international tournaments. Such approaches (requesting spiritual help and benediction) grant benign powers to older people. Yet, following the equation of sorcery (*kindoki*) with demonic activities, as occurs in many African urban centres, witchcraft accusations depict *the ndoki* as an evildoer, driven by jealousy, anger and hatred, and aspiring to destroy his/her opposition. These witchcraft accusations strongly manifest in social rejection of a particular individual. During interviews, I learned that the idea that 'all elders are *bandoki*' is rampant in Kinshasa, both among the young and among older people.[11] Although hardly any elderly person will actually agree that they are in fact *bandoki,* most of them will argue that other senior citizens 'must *have kindoki* inside them'. For the young, who are confronted with the early deaths of their siblings, friends and children, it seems unfair that older people are living longer. Often, older people are blamed for deaths in their streets. At best, these accusations are merely discursive; in other instances, seniors are insulted when they walk in the streets, or have stones thrown at their homes during the night, interrupting their sleep. Usually, the older people who have been subjected to witchcraft accusations told me, they didn't react to these accusations, but would respond that their old age is a blessing from God. 'If I really was a *ndoki*, the devil would have already gotten me long ago,' most of the older people reply.

Many Kinois, young and old, believe that the *homes de vieillards* house *bandoki*. For many urban residents, walking into a retirement home is a dangerous/risky event: it means visiting a group of people with supernatural powers. The residents of the *hospices*, on the other hand, usually deny such accusations about themselves, but will not refute the notion that fellow residents have occult powers or are practicing sorcery. During my research, one exception stood out. An elderly, disabled participant, unable to walk and confined to a wheel chair, told me that he had been a *nganga* during his 'valid' life, and that all his fellow *indigents* would consult him constantly to either trace lost goods or prolong their lives. His fellow residents, as well as the staff of his retirement home denied his confession, and encounters with this older person outside of the interview context made me wonder whether he was suffering from Alzheimer's or another mental affliction.

Often, older people joke about stereotypes of elders as *bandoki*, or else use it to achieve their own goals. On my very first visit to the retirement home of the Salvation Army (*Armée du Salut,* Kingabwa), one of the older women jokingly asked me if I wanted to hear about her latest trip in the shell of a groundnut, and how she nearly crashed her plane in Brussels. The idea of the retirement home as a den of witches and sorcerers is also shared by many elderly, who might use it to warn their children not to send them there and force them to continue taking care of their seniors. This is most poignantly illustrated by one of my (now late) female elderly participants, who continuously longed to go back to Kikwit (the city where she had lived for most of her married life), and who accused her children of not taking care of her. Her eldest and favourite child was living there. Her children in Kinshasa, who housed her, threatened to send her to a retirement home when they were tired of her requests to be sent back to Kikwit; to which she always responded that she would then become a *ndoki*, and each time that they visit her she would bewitch them as well.

Such discourse about being or becoming a *ndoki* shows that the idiom of witchcraft is central to the urban imagination about retirement homes. Yet, also significant is the discrepancy between the explanations given for why elderly people were living in retirement homes: most retirement home staff (themselves younger adults) stated that most of the residents had been chased away from their homes because of witchcraft accusations, while *the indigents* themselves usually gave very logical and reasonable explanations for their confinement to the retirement homes. None of them confirmed that they were labelled *as ndoki* and that this was the reason for their exclusion from the kin group. Rather, time and again, most older people referred to individual hardship, illness (mental illness, handicap), bad luck, cultural taboos (avoidance rules, see Obrist, Chapter Four), family conflicts, or 'temporary' situations to explain being in the retirement homes.[12] A case in point is Maman Mundele, a so-called *métisse* (mixed race person), who had been married to a Frenchman, but divorced him after giving him seven children. Her version is that one of her daughters brought her to the retirement home before she left for Angola, her husband's country of origin. Several of her children had died, Maman Mundele continued, while four were living in Europe. However, her only daughter still in Kinshasa, with whom she had been living, decided to look for new opportunities in Angola but could not take her elderly mother with her; and so brought her to the retirement home. According to the *home de vieillards* staff, three of her children were still living in Kinshasa but had accused Maman Mundele of being a *ndoki*. They brought her there three years ago and nobody had visited her since. I encountered many such contradictions. Older people, for their part, find completely logical justifications to explain why they are there. It seems easier to declare that one has no relatives rather than admit to having been accused of witchcraft.

Mobility of older people

'Old people should remain in their corners, and young ones ought to stay in their places, and so the young will respect their elders' (*Bavieux, il faut baza na coin na bango, bapetit il faut baza na place ya bango. Nde bapetit bakotosa bavieux*), said a participant during my research on youth and popular culture when I asked his opinion on 'fake old men', elderly people who emulate a youthful lifestyle, (Pype, 2012, 206). I repeat this quotation here for two reasons. First, the statement suggests an intimate connection between space and social age: where the young hang out, elderly people should not wander, and vice versa. The utterance also explicitly associates old age with immobility, yet this connection is not always accepted by all ageing Kinois. A greying woman (Lemba, 68 years old), who participated in weekly TV music shows where older people danced to Congolese urban music from the 1950s and 1960s, regretted that, '*bamibange batambolaka te, bafandaka na ndako*' (old people do not walk around, they just stay at home).

Commonly perceived, the lifeworlds of older people are characterised by rootedness, permanence and frozenness. Various explanations are at hand. First, most older people, especially when they become physically dependent, are stuck/confined at home and cannot move from the domestic space (see Obrist, Chapter Four). Second, cultural logics of respect firmly cement seniors in their dwelling. It is commonly understood that people with authority, elders and also the so-called 'big men' (Sg. *moto ya kilo*, successful businessmen, politicians, influential people), do not 'move' (see Pype, 2016). When older people wake up in the morning, it is the duty of the children and youth to go and see older people in their compounds, greet them and check that they are well. When visiting a compound, older people must be greeted first; one cannot expect an older person to get up and see the visitor. 'Big' and elderly people do not speak very much; they whisper, and they literally remain seated.[13] In such a context, immobility is a *sign* of power, honour and privilege, not the absence of these.

Yet, when one examines the places where elderly people actually lived before moving to their current residences, one notices that, despite cultural ideals of immobility, elderly people actually do move around often. Ageing Kinois, and in particular those whose caregiving is very demanding, are like urban nomads; they are sent from one (classificatory) child to another (see Obrist, Chapter Four). Older people with several children in Kinshasa are often sent from one household to the other. Most often, an older person is hosted by a child with fewer *charges*, that is to say expenses or burdens. Other children, who have many dependents, are spared taking in a parent. Most of my elderly participants had particular children or grandchildren with whom they preferred to stay, and it was very common for these names to be uttered, even when the hosting child was present during the interview.[14] Ageing women are most often sent to households with small babies, where the (classificatory) grandmothers can look after (and sometimes even nurse) the newborns. Often, when another daughter or daughter-in-law has given birth, the older woman moves to that household. On other occasions, conflicts among ageing individuals and residents (often following medical conditions or financial difficulties) result in older people being ousted, and having to look for another household.

Moving from one household to another is usually provoked by conflict. Many adults complain about their older people behaving like children (see also Freeman, Chapter Five), becoming capricious and extremely demanding, or else becoming too talkative, and sometimes even aggressive in their language and starting to physically attack others. On various occasions, I witnessed an elderly person literally slapping or spitting on grandchildren (usually teenagers). The grandchildren mostly take these attacks with a lot of humour. Despite the aggression, these interactions are often read as harmless, playful exchanges between identical classificatory groups because grandchildren and grandparents are structurally seen the same. In many vernacular languages of Congolese ethnic groups, the same word is used for both categories, for example, *bakoko* in Lingala. Yet, in daily life, these interactions place a significant burden on the harmony of the dwelling, often forcing the adult children to send their (classificatory) parent away.

Elderly people also complain about the care that their children provide (see also Van der Geest, Chapter One). The grievance I heard most often was that older people did not receive enough food; others complained of being ill and that relatives refused to take them to a doctor; smaller grievances included washing water being too cold. Often, these accusations were evoked before a conversation (or an informal interview) even started, thus seriously embarrassing the hosts who were often still around at the beginning of our conversations. According to many Kinois, Congolese older people are commonly given to jeremiads, expressing these sentiments wherever they go: to the priest, to the doctor, to the occasional visitor, in the shop, to a driver, and so on. This is also one of the reasons Kinois prefer to keep their elderly relatives at home and isolate them, in an effort not to stain their reputation and not to be called 'bad children' (Li. Sg. *mwana mabe*).

Usually the adult children decide among themselves what to do with an ageing parent, and the move is often undertaken without the elderly person being consulted (at best, he or she is informed). The case of Maman Mosa echoes many stories I collected about older people's housing conditions. When I met Maman Mosa in August 2011 (she died a few months later), she was living in Mbanza-Lemba with her classificatory grandson, his wife and their children. Nobody really knew her age; she herself claimed to be almost 100 and maintained that she was born 'on the day that sugar entered into Congo'. According to her relatives, Maman Mosa was in her late 80s. She had only arrived in Kinshasa three years earlier, having spent her entire life in Maniema. She found herself without any children, living with her sister until the latter died. Her brother's children met Maman Mosa when they travelled to Maniema for the funeral of their paternal aunt. They convinced her to come with them to Kinshasa. Although initially reluctant, Maman Mosa gave in and found herself living in Kinshasa. Yet, her life in Kinshasa has been very mobile: in these three years, she moved among her deceased brother's grandchildren, never staying more than six months in the same compound. She lived in three different municipalities of Kinshasa (Matete, Kasa-Vubu and Limete), and at the end found herself in Mbanza-Lemba. All the other households accused her of being a *ndoki*, but Maman Pauline, her final host, did not believe these accusations. She joked that she had never seen Maman Mosa in the night; but she did report that life with Maman Mosa was extremely hard. As Maman Pauline told us, Maman Mosa defecated everywhere in the house, insulted her caretakers, and constantly quarrelled in a quite childlike fashion with Maman Pauline's children, who are between two and eight years old. In addition, Maman Mosa was a Muslim, while her relatives were Christians. The difference in religious attachments might also have contributed to the witchcraft accusations expressed by her Christian classificatory children. In addition, although Maman Mosa received 1000FC (US$1) every morning from her (classificatory) grandson, with which she could buy a soda or dried meat, she begged in the street, thus harming her hosts' reputations, and was perceived as a troublemaker by her younger relatives.

While Maman Mosa accepted each move, other elderly participants at times disagreed when they were sent away. Usually, however, ageing individuals are powerless and have to accept their guardians' decisions.[15] Maman Mosa was someone who could easily have been sent to a retirement home.

Housing matters

As discussed in this volume's introduction, who houses whom matters in terms of the construction and evaluation of care. In Kinshasa too, who houses whom, and who shares the same living space with whom, orient practices of care. Yet, these practices are likewise fundamentally structured by social rules and restraints. Particular ethnic groups, like the Luba, but also the Chokwe and Pende, impose the rule that (classificatory) mothers-in-law cannot share living spaces with their sons-in-law. Virilocality and neolocality are the main strategies for respecting this avoidance obligation. Yet, when a mother-in-law becomes ill or can no longer live in her home, or when she arrives in the city and her daughter is the only relative who has space, then, if the family is wealthy, the mother-in-law will usually be housed in an *annexe*, a small room behind the main house. Often the elderly woman will also have her own washing facilities. The reason that participants gave for this arrangement is to avoid the mother-in-law and son-in-law (both *bokilo* in Lingala) seeing each other's nudity. This avoidance rule is taken seriously by all parties;[16] and mystical punishments, such as infertility, illness and death, are said to follow such taboo violations.

In a city like Kinshasa, where housing facilities depend on one's wealth, housing a mother-in-law in a separate building is a luxury, unaffordable to many. Many of Kinshasa's retirement homes' female residents who still have relatives living in the city, are there because of lack of space in their daughters' houses, and because the avoidance rule must be respected. One could argue that these cultural taboos function as cultural codes for imposing respect among the various positions in a family group, and restrict conflict potentials between people with shared interests (interest in the affection of the married woman, as a daughter and as a wife); indeed, all of my female participants explicitly mentioned this taboo as the main reason for why they were where they were, and accepted that fate.[17] While these taboos operate among many Congolese ethnic groups, the mystical punishment is said to be strongest among the Luba; thus explaining why most female *indigents* are either of Luba descent, or have a daughter who married into a Luba family.

Photo 2.2: A rare mural painting orienting towards a retirement home (© Katrien Pype, 2013)

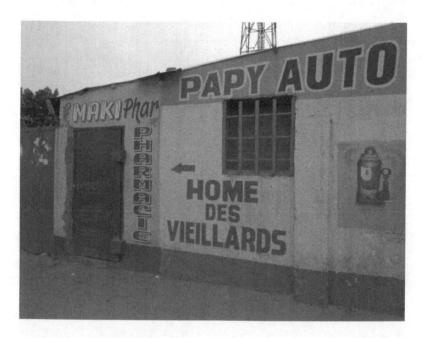

Becoming an *indigent*

Despite the ethnic–related taboos, *ideally* Kinshasa's elderly people live among their relatives until they die. As in many other African settings, family relationships, especially ties with children, are the basic social spaces of care provision for older people. Therefore, unsurprisingly, most of the *indigents* (male and female) have no children of their own. Several of these female *indigents* had been married, yet had not been able to conceive. Very often, these women had been the first spouses of a polygamous man, who then entered into a second marriage in order to father children. In all cases, the first wife would be supported until the death of her husband; but after his death, the man's children would not feel obliged to feed and host their mother's rival. Usually, these older women without offspring lived with several of their siblings' children, although, often, following the siblings' deaths, the classificatory children would start neglecting the elder in their compound.

Yet, in an urban context, equally important to family relations are the social contacts that individuals establish outside the family (compare Van Eeuwijk, Chapter Three and De Klerk, Chapter Six). The *réseau* (Pype, 2012, 91) refers to broader and less permanent networks and connections that construct and mediate a sense of belonging in the urban environment. These are temporary relations and do not always lead to clearly profiled social groups with public identities or genealogies (Pype, 2012, 65). Kinois persistently attempt to connect with others in temporary ways, without necessarily obtaining firm social positions in the lives of these 'contacts'. Still, these are said to be important connections for physical, social and economic survival. Some elderly people are able to rely on these contacts for long periods of time. However, in the end, the ties with these connections (who themselves belong to firmer social groups in which they have their own obligations) are too weak to provide sufficient care for older people. As a result, most retirement home residents have socially become non-persons within the (larger) family, and are bereft of viable social relations (*contacts*) outside the family group.

Catholic churches provide the first alternative support network for older people outside the family or informal support groups. Various female and male *indigents* have been hosted for a while by non-related fellow Catholic church members. Usually, these stays are short, as they depend on the host's financial and material capacities. Older people would then often be totally abandoned, seeing no other way than asking the church for help to live in a retirement home. Some might sleep in the church compound for a few days in the hope that another fellow church member would agree to take them.

On Thursday evenings, all over the city, *CVB* (Cellule de Base)[18] groups meet, either in the homes of fellow Catholics or in church compounds. These small prayer units are organised according to geography, bringing together members who live in the same neighbourhood. Prayers and Bible readings during these weekly meetings provide constant spiritual renewal for Catholic church members, but they also serve as social surveillance systems. At the end of the CVB meetings, participants are asked to name individuals in the neighbourhood who are in need of material and/or financial assistance (not limited to older people). Usually, a small group of CVB members then visits the needy individuals once a week on Sundays; they pray with older people, read sections of the Bible, keep them company, and provide them with basic items like soap, and some food and medicine, paid for by local CVB members. Here, the family is not the basis of caring activities – rather, a Christian ethos that incorporates all individuals within the universal body of the 'children of God' (spiritual family) pushes Catholics to reach out to people in need. Older people are then not cared for as *bakoko* (family elders) but instead acquire the status of *babola* (people in need). Rather than the intergenerational contract (see Freeman, Chapter Five and Hoffman, Chapter Seven), it is the individual's obligation towards the Christian God that drives feeding, clothing and providing company to older people.

In certain instances, CVB members alert the priest or the municipal social affairs office about needing to intervene in the living conditions of older people. The 'official' route to becoming an *indigent* is to obtain an *attestation d'indigence*. This document can only be acquired after the municipal administration (at the Town Hall)[19] has sent social workers to the ageing person's family. Based on their investigations into the economic and affective possibilities of the family, social workers write an official report of destituteness (*procès-verbal de constat d'état d'indigence or a pv de constat d'indigence pour les soins médicaux*). This report needs to be approved by the city authorities, who then decide whether and where to place the old man or woman, who, through this document has officially become an 'indigent person'.[20] Once recognised as an *indigent*, one is *ideally* under the care of the Congolese state (compare with Van der Geest, Chapter One). In practice, this means that state agents (social workers at the Town Hall) try to find a bed in a *hospice* for the *indigent*. An *indigent* is officially declared to be without relatives, whereupon his or her care is assured by the state. Here, *indigents* are cared for as 'citizens'. Notwithstanding the role played by the Catholic Church or its emissaries in the acceptance of elderly people into retirement homes, being an *indigent* is in the very first place a civic identity, tested and validated by state employees.

Very often, CVB members or other religious figures see to the administrative work, contact the municipal authorities, and ensure the transfer of an individual to a *hospice*. Sometimes, elderly people move directly from the hospital to the retirement home. Such was the case for Papa Misho, a man in his early 70s, who arrived at the *St Pierre* retirement home after suffering from thrombosis in 2005. By that time, he had already left his second wife, with whom he had three sons. His first wife had died in the village, decades earlier. His children from 'the first bed' (first marriage) had grown up in the village, and he was largely out of touch with them. The man had also fathered three other children with different women in Kinshasa, in Brazzaville and in Pointe Noire. His second wife told me she left Papa Misho because of his infidelity and prolonged absences from home. When Papa Misho fell ill, his (now late) brother took him to the largest hospital in the city, Maman Yemo. Papa Misho rarely received any visits while there and could not afford to pay his bills. After six months, the Catholic nurses of the hospital brought the man to a retirement home. The hospital bed needed to be free for new, paying patients. Papa Misho knew the names of his children residing in Kinshasa and their exact addresses. He even knew that his ex-wife had told their sons that he had died. Still, every morning and night, he prayed to God that his children would come and find him. Papa Misho did not undertake any effort to reach the children himself because they were too small in his opinion – they were in their late teens and were not yet independent, so he could not ask them to take care of him. Still, he had hopes that he would see his children again. But, his hopes were not that they would take him in. He had accepted that he would die in that/a retirement home.

While Papa Misho could not control his transfer and thus was totally bereft of any agency, other elderly people do act as agents (see Caplan, 1998), and, as long as their mental capacities are still functioning, they are able to influence their social space. An interesting example is the case discussed above, where a female participant threatened to bewitch her children were she sent to a retirement home. Yet, in other instances, it is older people themselves who choose to leave the household and live in a *hospice*. Various men (never women) made personal requests at the town hall to be identified as *indigent* and be placed in a *home*.

Papa José, now 94 years old, entered a state retirement home in September 2012 after a conflict with his grandchildren, who had sold his compound. As an 'old combatant' (he had fought in the Second World War), Papa José had received a house in the municipality of Bandalungwa in the early 1960s in reward from the state for his deeds during the war. He had 11 children with his wife, who passed away two years earlier at home after a long illness. By the early 2000s, three of his children had died, and the others were living abroad. He had several grandchildren in Kinshasa, some of whom stayed with him in Bandalungwa; others scattered throughout the city after they had set up their own households. In June 2012, Papa José overheard his grandchildren scheming to sell his compound. A few days later, they sent the priest to convince him of moving into a retirement home. For a few months, Papa José resisted, but as he became more and more angry with his grandchildren, he decided he no longer wanted to live with them. He asked the Catholic priest for help, and went on his own to the town hall to request an attestation of *indigence*. Joined by the Catholic priest, he went into the *hospice* and told his grandchildren he did not want to see them. They are supposed to wait until he calls them and invites them.

I collected several narratives of old men who still had relatives living in the city, and who were in good health but resided in a *hospice*. In these cases, serious disagreements with their children or grandchildren pushed them to abandon the family home; in all cases, they have forbidden their offspring to visit them.

To conclude this section, I would like to draw attention to the politics of the word *indigent*. As noted above, this identity is officially granted by the state – conferred on people who need to be cared for by the state. There are other kinds of *indigents*, such as orphans who are sent to state-run orphanages. However, the English word *indigent* refers to an impoverished individual.[21] Here, no notion of state intervention is included in the semantics. It is the Lingala word *babola* that takes on the precise meaning of poverty. *Babola* are not necessarily elderly people, but can also be impoverished widows, people living on the streets, and so on. In the Kinois context, talking about *babola* suggests an activation of solidarity. Within Catholic circles, then, the word *babola* is more commonly used than *indigent* and addresses responsibilities within the religious community (see above).

Caring benefactors

From time to time, the *indigents* are visited by 'strangers' who may donate a bag of rice, medicine or clothes.[22] Feeding, clothing, providing health care are familiar care activities, but in the context of the retirement home, these practices occur outside the family group or the informal support group. Usually, visits by *bienfaiteurs* (benefactors), as these strangers are called by the retirement homes' staff and residents, follow a predictable pattern: the donor presents him- or herself to the retirement home's central office, gives the food and pharmaceuticals to the staff, and spends some time with older people, usually praying and making small talk.

Sometimes, these individuals have been visiting for years, yet no intense relationships are being forged between older people and the sponsor. At times, some *indigents* might know the names of their benefactors, but they do not have their phone numbers, nor can they transmit requests. Donations are usually made in an anonymous way without becoming personal. This shows that for the benefactors, the recipients are not seen as individuals with personal histories, rather they are receivers because of their identity as residents of the retirement home.

Representatives of small-scale entrepreneurs, international corporations like mobile phone companies and even the presidency donate goods (clothes, pharmaceuticals, food) and money to retirement home staff and the *indigents* themselves. Motivations of these offerings differ according to the donors. While such gifts are necessary for the daily functioning of the retirement homes (I have been told that without these gifts, there would hardly be any food), these contributions are the manifestations of various kinds of intentions, where older people are given pivotal roles in the acknowledgement or purification of wealth and power.

Although, from the perspective of the *indigents*, these gifts appear improvised, donations are structured according to laws specific to the religious, corporate and international human rights worlds, in which retirement homes become symbolic spaces where the wealthy convert their economic and symbolic capital into 'good' wealth and power.

Most small-scale entrepreneurs whose donations I mentioned above, were Catholics, and, unsurprisingly made reference to the tenth Biblical Commandment. One such donor, Mère Justine, is a successful female entrepreneur. She often travels to China and Dubai, where she buys household utensils for resale in Kinshasa's largest market. Mère Justine also manages a small hotel and bar in Mont Ngafula, one of Kinshasa's municipalities. Here, lovers can rent a room for a few hours. In the popular imagination, hotels are commonly regarded as immoral, because such spaces are known as spaces where sex out of wedlock takes place. Unsurprisingly, from a Christian point of view, this woman's wealth is 'bad money' (*mbongo mabe*). Every three months, Mère Justine buys soap, bags of rice and shirts for a total amount of 10 per cent of what she has made during that time, and takes these goods, along with some cash, to a retirement home. At times, she donates more than US$1,000, at other times she spends up to US$3,000. By offering a part of her wealth, this business woman purifies it; she gives a tenth of her monthly income to God's needy, and thus turns herself into a good Christian subject. 'God will bless me,' she told me during an informal interview.

When querying the residents in the *hospices* about the potential spiritual effects of these gifts (which are regarded as coming from 'bad money'), their replies were very pragmatic: on the one hand because they regard themselves as Christians, they claim that they are well protected against any bad spiritual effects that such gifts could bring; on the other hand, there was an elaborate explanation as to why these gifts would not bring any harm: the contributions manifest the acceptance of God's power. Sponsoring older people is like giving to God: God obviously likes these elderly people, otherwise they would not be blessed with such longevity; therefore the givers' intentions at the time of the giving were, according to most of the receivers, already pure and Christian, and so without detrimental effect.

Larger international companies such as breweries, mobile phone companies, and food producers also sponsor retirement homes. These donations are part of their corporate social responsibilities, according to international conventions that force companies to redistribute a percentage of their revenues within the societies where they are making their profits. While the Congolese entertainment industry (music, TV shows, football) benefits most from this support, retirement homes also gain. Gifts from these larger corporations are made at regular intervals: just before Christmas and on 1 October. The timing of these donations is not accidental. The pre-Christmas gifts are embedded in the local tax regulations (before year end); and those made on 1 October are embedded within international human rights policies: the UN declared 1 October as International Day of Older Persons in order to raise awareness of issues affecting older people, such as senescence and abuse of elderly people. Older people are invisible in corporate marketing materials disseminated all over Kinshasa, yet, in the case of mobile phone companies, for example, senior citizens are addressed in the *Vodacoeur* ('the heart of Vodacom') and *Airtel et les Gens* ('Airtel and the People') programmes of the mobile phone companies' charity funds. In these programmes, older people figure alongside orphans and widows. Network personnel regularly visit retirement homes and donate food and material goods (mattresses, clothes, soap, and so on).

Local politicians are a third category of benefactors. Here, the goal is to gain the affection of the public and approval as a politician. Recently (since 2007) international NGOs have rediscovered Kinshasa's retirement homes. Money collected in Europe is spent on painting walls and building new beds and closets for older people.

Very often, these donation activities are public events: cameras are in tow, and journalists are invited to witness and report on these visits. On the local TV stations, one often sees video reports of visits from companies and politicians to these *hospices*. Usually, older people are not interviewed – they are merely the décor for the event. The images show donors addressing television audiences and retirement home staff. In late December 2012, the first lady, Olive Kalembe, visited seven of Kinshasa's eight retirement homes. During Maman Olive's visits to the *homes de vieillards,* various cameras filmed her cleaning toilets, helping in the kitchen, and talking with the *indigents* in their rooms. The propaganda focused on maternal tasks and donations: at state-run retirement homes the first lady gave each resident a piece of cloth, milk powder, sugar, manioc powder, medicine and an envelope containing US$50; at privately managed homes, she donated half of those amounts. Here, as in the visual reports of companies' visits to *hospices*, older people are talked *about* and represented as 'people in need'. In these charity clips, they are defined as sick, hungry and in need of decent clothing; the retirement home, just like the orphanage and the hospital, has become the exemplary décor for these practices.

This particular staging of the residents, of the *indigent*s, as lacking any voice, opinion, or experience, suggests that the media reports on donations have a value different from the anonymous donations made by individuals who merely want to purchase God's blessing. I suggest that by publicly donating to the city's needy, and thus staging themselves as 'good Christians', the wealthy and powerful are deliberately trying to obtain collective approval from the larger Kinois community (who is witnessing the gift giving). Here, the retirement home occupies a symbolic position for the city's wealthy – it functions as the Other of the lifeworlds of the rich and the famous, one whose existence is necessary for the wealthy to maintain their power. Yet, all of these performances of care are situated outside of familial or informal support groups, and instead are embedded within other structures of reciprocity: exchanges with the divine/the Congolese state/the market.

Social exclusion done and undone

Retirement homes, although fairly small in number, offer invaluable material on the ways in which Kinois deal with their senior citizens, about how the urban and national authorities approach the city's senior population, and even suggest a great deal about the imaginations of older people at large. Even though retirement homes have thus far been invisible in the academic literature on African societies, they occupy particular symbolic spaces within the urban imagination at large. In the context of Kinshasa, they are at times remnants of colonisation and evoke foreign practices of caring for older people; in other instances, they become extremely localised, especially when identified as the spaces of witches, or when benefactors make their donations. Retirement homes are also very local spaces when they are intervened upon by their immediate surroundings: by children who come and fetch water, or as elderly residents attempt to make money by engaging in petty trade just outside.

Kinshasa's *homes de vieillards* are spaces of social exclusion, mostly housing elderly people without familial support, where exogenous practices of care are enacted. This social interpretation of the retirement home represents an African appropriation of the facility. The oldest retirement homes were established by the Belgian colonial government to accommodate elderly colonial residents or their local staff. The English concept of *retirement home* suggests a modern, political-economic approach towards the life course according to which elderly people retire, literally withdraw from society. Related to the concept of the 'retirement home' is the verb 'to retire', which is now commonly understood as withdrawing from the economy and no longer contributing to the state economy. Such a view of the *home de vieillards* and its residents is unwarranted in Kinshasa, where the formal economy scarcely functions, not because the state is barely able to fulfil its role as provider of basic care, but because most of these homes' residents (with the exception of the women who are there because of cultural taboos) are excluded (willingly or not) from their families and have thus lost their identities in the primary space of identity attribution: the family.

When reading the embedment of retirement homes in the urban society, and in particular when examining the interactions between 'the city' and residents of retirement homes, however, we see that these *indigents* have acquired surprising meanings, and a different kind of value. And this is probably one of the most fundamental aspects of caring: showing that people's lives matter and have meaning for others. By being recognised and addressed as people who can pray for others or receive gifts, older people are ascribed good intentions, and, what is more important, an essential role in urban society.

Notes

[1] President Kabila's plan to 'modernise the country' (*la révolution de la modernité*) – which started in 2006 – includes the construction of two new retirement homes. At the time of finalising this chapter, the constructions had not yet begun.

[2] 'Care' here is defined as an assemblage of emotional and technical/practical performances (Van der Geest, 2002, 8): relating to the manifestation of concern, dedication and attachment on the one hand, and carrying out activities for others who, for physical or emotional reasons, are unable to do so (for example, feeding, washing, housing people).

[3] Names have been changed to guarantee privacy.

[4] From that moment, they receive a (symbolic) pension every three months.

[5] This paragraph comes from Pype (2012, 205–6).

[6] Many Kinois claim that Papa Wemba is older. He supposedly lies about his age to keep a more youthful appearance.

[7] Being called 'vieux' still remains something many young adults long for, because of the normative practices it entails: deference, public display of respect, and authority. The idea of 'vieux' is very much a gendered, masculine notion.

[8] In one of the retirement homes, where residents do not have to sell in order to be able to procure additional food and medicine because all of that is fairly well provided, a female resident still sells cigarettes outside and inside the retirement home. The profits she makes are sent to her daughter. She feels obliged to help her offspring in any way she can [this woman is in a retirement home due to social taboos, see pp 55–56].

[9] The Lingala verb kobokola (to nurture) is at times used in talking about providing care for older people. However, the verb is mainly used in the context of nurturing small children.

[10] Many of these associations also turn into rotating savings and credit associations (ristourne/likelemba). Participation in a rotating savings and credit association is expensive, and not all elderly can afford this. Most informants who were saving money in that way claimed to be doing it in order to guarantee a good funeral for themselves. Older people do not fully count on their relatives for a good funeral, and try to raise debts among their peers, who also will have to contribute to their own funerals.

[11] Colleagues working in other parts of Africa have observed the same phenomenon. There also seems to be a gender bias: elderly women are more vulnerable to witchcraft accusations (Mary, 1987; Meudec, 2009). We should also raise the question of how this is biased by demographic realities (women living longer than men).

[12] Interviews with state officials confirm that witchcraft accusations, as the main reason for the transfer of older people to retirement homes, are only relevant in a very small number of cases.

[13] This symbolic approach to the embodiment of social power and authority also encourages an older person to send someone to make the phone call on his or her behalf (Pype, 2016).

[14] Most of my elderly female participants who were still in good physical health tried to contribute to the hosting household by either looking after children, preparing food, cleaning and sometimes selling items like groundnuts, soft drinks and other small articles. Revenue from these commercial activities is small but symbolic, as it shows caregivers that older people are willing to contribute. In the case of senior men, I did not observe these kinds of activities.

[15] Very often it is the adult children who decide to bring their ageing parent(s) over to Kinshasa. They make all travel arrangements, sometimes without the parent even being informed. Those older people who only arrive in Kinshasa at an advanced age, in particular, are totally dependent on their children, as they have not acquired the skills to navigate in a megalopolis and sometimes do not speak Lingala, the city's vernacular language.

[16] One of the male research participants, a man in his early 50s living in Kikwit, told me with much amusement about how his wife's paternal aunt, so his classificatory mother-in-law, was staying for two weeks in his house, for the duration of her visit to the city. Usually, he left the house rather early; his mother-in-law would wash herself only after he had left. One morning, he had not gone to work, and while talking to his wife, he saw her mother only wearing a piece of cloth in the hallway. She was on her way to the bathroom but had to pass through the eating area. Shocked, because she had not expected her son-in-law to be at home, she turned slowly and walked, pushing herself against the wall, back to her room. Her behaviour, literally fleeing, shows how inappropriate it was for her to pass by her son-in-law only half covered.

[17] Unsurprisingly, these women usually had visitors (their daughters and grandchildren).

[18] Related to these CVB groups are the *bureaux ya caritasi*, which are structures operating at a higher level in the Catholic Church. Here, people are not visited in their houses but rather in hospital.

[19] Kinshasa has 24 municipalities, each of them with their own mayor and town hall.

[20] In 2011, there were 12 requests for placement in retirement homes, with only two older people able to move into a *home*. Becoming an *indigent* recognised by the state is the official route. It is clear that there are many more elderly people moving around, and the Ministry of Social Affairs is not always involved in the allocation of places in retirement homes run by the Catholic Church.

[21] See the Oxford English dictionary: 'indigent' as a noun refers to 'an indigent person; one poor and needy' (online edition).

[22] During interviews, staff of retirement homes complained about no longer receiving *mpiodi* (fish) or trousers for their *indigents*. These goods are apparently more costly. While donated food and pharmaceuticals are usually managed by retirement home staff, the clothes are kept by the older people themselves. Often, in their closets (if there are any) or next to his or her bed, an *indigent* person has a plastic bag which contains – depending on the duration of their stay in the retirement home – a large number of shirts, still in their plastic wrappings.

Acknowledgements

I would like to acknowledge the help of Marie-Jeanne Musito, who assisted me during visits to retirement homes. This research would also have been impossible without the hospitality of staff and residents at the retirement homes, as well as their relatives. Social workers and state employees at the town halls of Lemba and Bandalungwa, and staff at the Ministries of Public Health and of Social Affairs have provided invaluable data. This chapter has also benefited much from conversations with the Kongo and Muhunga families. I would also particularly like to thank Florence Nzeba and Amitié Lukesa for their companionship during this research. VLIR-UOS funding through the University of Antwerp and a Marie Curie postdoctoral fellowship (PIOF-GA-2009-252331) made this research possible.

References

Alber, E, Van der Geest, S, Whyte, SR (eds), 2008, *Generations in Africa: Connections and conflicts*, Münster: LIT Verlag

Aguilar, MI, 1998, *The politics of age and gerontocracy in Africa: Ethnographies of the past and memories of the present*, Trenton, NJ: Africa World Press

Caplan, P (ed), 1998, *Risk revisited*, London: Pluto Press

Christiansen, C, Utas, M, Vigh, H (eds), 2008, *Navigating youth, generating adulthood. Social becoming in an African context*, Uppsala: Nordiska Afrika institutet

Cole, J, Durham, D (eds), 2007, *Generations and globalization: Youth, age, and family in the new world economy*, Bloomington, IN: Indiana University Press

Durham, D, 2000, Introduction: Youth and the social imagination in Africa, *Anthropological Quarterly* 73, 3, 113–20

Hareven, T, 1996, *Aging and generational relations: Life-course and cross-cultural perspectives*, New York: De Gruyter

Honwana, A, De Boeck, F (eds), 2005, *Makers and breakers: Children and youth in postcolonial Africa*, Oxford: James Currey

Hurwicz, M-L, 1995, Introduction: Anthropology, aging, and health, *Medical Anthropology Quarterly*, 9, 2, 143–45

Keith, J, 1980, "The best is yet to be": Toward an anthropology of age, *Annual Review of Anthropology* 9, 339–64

Lamb, S, 2000, *White saris and sweet mangoes: Aging, gender and body in North India*, Berkeley: University of California Press

Makoni, S, Stroeken, K, 2002, *Ageing in Africa: Linguistic and anthropological approaches*, Farnham: Ashgate

Mary, A, 1987, Sorcellerie bocaine, sorcellerie africaine: le social, le symbolique et l'imaginaire, Cahiers du LASA, *Laboratoire De Sociologie Anthropologique De l'Université de Caen* 7, 124–52

Meudec, M, 2009, Éthique pragmatique de la recherche anthropologique, le cas d'une étude de l'obea h à Ste-Lucie, *Cahiers de Recherches Sociologiques*, 48, 155–74

Myerhof, B, 1978, *Number our days*, New York, London, Toronto, Sydney, Tokyo, Singapore: Simon and Schuster

Obrist, B, Van Eeuwijk, P, Weiss, M, 2003, Health anthropology and urban health research, *Anthropology and Medicine* 10, 3, 267–74

Pype, K, 2012, *The making of the Pentecostal melodrama: Religion, media, and gender in Kinshasa*, Oxford/New York: Berghahn Books

Pype, K, 2016, Brokers of belonging: Elders and intermediaries in Kinshasa's mobile phone culture, in W Mano, W Willems (eds) *Everyday Media Culture in Africa: Audiences and Users*, London: Routledge (in press)

Pype, K, 2017, Dancing on the rhythm of Léopoldville: Nostalgia, urban critique and intergenerational differences in Kinshasa's TV music shows, *Journal of African Cultural Studies*, http://dx.doi.org/1 0.1080/13696815.2016.1189816

Sokolovsky, J (ed), 1997, *The cultural contexts of aging* (2nd ed), Westport, CT: Greenwood

Spencer, P, (ed), 1990, *Anthropology and the riddle of the Sphinx: Paradoxes of change in the life course*, London: Routledge, ASA Monographs, 28

Van der Geest, S, 1997, Money and respect: The changing value of old age in rural Ghana, *Africa: Journal of the International African Institute* 76, 4, 534–59

Van der Geest, S, 2002, Respect and reciprocity: Care of elderly people in rural Ghana, *Journal of Cross-Cultural Gerontology* 17, 3–31

Van Eeuwijk, P, Obrist, B (eds), 2006, *Vulnerabilität, Migration und Altern: Medizinethnologische Ansätzeim Spannungsfeld von Theorie und Praxis.* Zürich: Seismo Verlag

Older people providing care for older people in Tanzania: against conventions – but accepted

Peter van Eeuwijk

Introduction: older people as care providers

The ageing and care interface in Sub-Saharan African contexts has not yet been extensively investigated. Moreover, care provision for older Africans requires further understanding in terms of its quantitative and qualitative dimensions. In particular, intra- and intergenerational care provision, where older people provide care to other older people is still largely under-researched. This contribution outlines how such care practices and arrangements in Tanzania occur and affect old-age vulnerability in relation to health and illness; and how both older caregivers and care-receivers navigate within and between social spaces in circumstances of critical health moments.

From the perspective of an older person who needs support, old-age vulnerability is strongly shaped by the presence or absence of care provision (Van Eeuwijk, 2006b). Normative attitudes and views in most societies assign the provision of care to younger generations, and in particular to women (Bongaarts and Zimmer, 2002; Whyte et al, 2008; Sokolovsky, 2009). This picture is embedded in ideal or idealised imaginations based on, for example, kinship relations, filial piety and generational responsibility, gender roles, family solidarity, religious obligations and moral reciprocity, and professional ethics (Van Eeuwijk, 2014). Yet, real care practices show that older people – and to a great extent older women – also implement, govern and maintain care provision. Old-age vulnerability in relation to the ambivalent social valuation of 'good care' or 'bad care' certainly builds on these culturally shaped normative and ideal premises (Mol et al, 2010). Care provided by older people for older people does not meet social expectations, does not comply, to a great extent, with normative attitudes and is often construed as a transgression or implicit violation of these meaningful social and cultural codes. In other words, older care-receivers are thought to have become more vulnerable with regard to care and health as a result of the increased vulnerability of their aged carers.

Generally, older people as caregivers are no longer a rare or uncommon phenomenon in the social sciences. Many studies on ageing, health and care in low- and middle-income countries show that, because of major societal transformations, such as demographic and epidemiologic transitions, social transformations, change of lifestyle, migration and urbanisation, older people increasingly assume roles of major caregivers in their households. In particular, research on HIV/AIDS in Sub-Saharan Africa (for example Ssengonzi, 2009; Ardington et al, 2010; Ogunmefun et al, 2011; De Klerk, 2011; also see De Klerk, Chapter Six) has revealed an important transformation in care practice, namely the shift from older care-receivers to older care providers for HIV-infected spouses, AIDS-diseased children and orphaned grandchildren. For some time now, non-governmental organisations (such as HelpAge International) and multilateral organisations have emphasised the growing importance of older people as caregivers in African households, and have asked for more recognition and support for them (WHO, 2002; HelpAge International, 2004; 2012; EveryChild and HelpAge International, 2012). Still, older people acting as major caregivers, particularly for other elderly individuals, whether in intra- and intergenerational, informal and formal, care relationships – including non-kin institutionalised eldercare – represent a new issue in social science research on ageing, health and care. As such, this questions the centrality of the immediate family in care activities (see Hoffman, Chapter Seven) and is associated with changing social spaces and the transgression of moral principles. At the same time it remains widely underestimated and under-researched.

This chapter provides insight into the 'elder for elder' care phenomenon by examining four facets of this particular care arrangement, and explores the quality of the social spaces interconnected with this kind of care relationship:

- varieties of care arrangements with older people as major caregivers;
- care activities performed by these older care providers and the burdens they carry;
- extended care arrangements in critical or problematic health situations;
- non-kin care provided by older people in institutions.

The author approaches the subject from a social agency angle, which older caregivers may develop in order to reduce or mitigate the burden of eldercare. The agentic extension of social space in problematic caregiving moments may well contest normative expectations of care and transgress norms and values, but it can also reaffirm kinship relations (Van Eeuwijk, 2011; Gerold, 2013). Schnegg et al (2010, 25–6) argue that generational tensions between structures accrued from rules and norms, and their subsequent transgression, finally lead to societal transformations, which in turn creates new options for both actions and spaces in the relationships between and within generations.

Research setting and methodology

This study refers to older people, their social spaces and their physical environments at three different research[1] sites in Tanzania. The main sites are multi-ethnic and -religious Dar es Salaam (Temeke Municipality, Ward Mbagala and *Mta* Mbagala), the country's largest city, a rural town (Ikwiriri *Kusini*/South Ikwiriri), and a small remote village (Bumba, consisting of two hamlets) in Rufiji District (Coast Region). The great majority of the study sites' inhabitants are Muslim *Warufiji* ('people from Rufiji') because the given research setting investigates the rural–urban ties of this ethnic group exclusively (Gerold, 2012; 2013; Simon, 2012; see also Obrist, Chapter Four).

The study setting includes different societal levels, namely:

• a community study;
• a household study;
• an age cohort study.

The main criteria for participation in this study are:

• a household with at least one older person;
• this person being 60 years or older.

The lower age limit for inclusion in our study (60 years[2]) corresponds to the official definition of Tanzania's 'National Ageing Policy' issued in 2003 (Ministry of Labour, Youth Development and Sports, 2003).

The study uses a combination of quantitative research methods (such as statistics and structured questionnaires), qualitative techniques (in-depth interviews, focus group discussions, direct observation and case studies), and documentary instruments (photo and film documentation) (Gerold, 2012; Simon, 2012).

The above-mentioned broader community study involves, among others, one particular question about the role and burden of older caregivers. The main empirical data for this chapter derive from the household study and are complemented by selected qualitative evidence from the community and the age cohort study.

The research on institutionalised eldercare provided by older people results, for the most part, from the additional activities of team members in the field. Smaller, less formalised institutions such as clubs, associations, and, to some degree, self-help groups, are located within particular research areas in Dar es Salaam and Rufiji District. The researchers have come across non-kin corporations in the course of their daily fieldwork, meeting them through institutional activities or by acquiring personal information from other older people. The non-governmental organisations and the formal eldercare institutions are partly identified by team members in their study areas (for Zanzibar and Dar es Salaam) and partly suggested by Dar es Salaam-based HelpAge International Tanzania, followed by further internet research (for Dar es Salaam and Zanzibar, and for additional study sites Arusha and Moshi). These latter institutions can be visited by personal appointment, and in some cases also by showing an official permit. These visits include not only formal meetings and talks with mostly older board members, directors and managers, but also a short informal oral exchange (including photo documentation) with older people who live in these institutions or receive homecare support from them. Most informal groups such as an older men's club based at the local market, or an association with income-generating activities, allow a researcher to be present and observe their ongoing activities. Team members also conduct semi-structured interviews with selected older group members.

Care and eldercare

Multiple ambiguities, such as emotional/technical, caregiving/care-receiving, attitude/activity, affection/work and burden/relief characterise and shape notions of 'care'. Keeping these intrinsic opacities, overlaps and polarisations in mind, the concept of 'eldercare' epitomises the ways in which a society – oscillating between cultural representations, moral claims, structural principles and practical necessities – concerns itself with its vulnerable older people and supports them in times of need (Tronto, 2009; Van Eeuwijk, 2006a; 2006b; 2007; 2011).

The understanding of 'care' as both a relational and temporal concept (Kleinman, 2009; Kleinman and Van der Geest, 2009) has also shaped the study setting of our research on 'ageing, health and care' in Tanzania. An initial and broader approach situates care as a social and cultural practice, and thus a relational phenomenon, examining what it means to be related to a (frail) person in need of support. The second (more narrow) analysis clarifies care as interpersonal assistance, or interference, on the occasion of an individual's critical and problematic (health) moments. Both perspectives frame this chapter's four elder-to-elder care dimensions. Care as social practice and relational occurrence in everyday life refers to:

• compositions of care arrangements with older people as both major care providers and care-receivers (see Table 3.1);
• care activities provided by older caregivers for aged people (Table 3.2);
• provision of care and support for older people in care institutions.

Care as concrete interference at critical moments, however, relates to the extension of care arrangements in problematic (health) situations and, in this way, to the expansion of social spaces, including old and new kinship relations (Table 3.3), and institutionalised non-kin care provision.

Particular attention is drawn to the capacity of older caregivers to shape their responsiveness to problematic situations, such as chronic frailty or degenerative health impairments, as well as intensive care and immediate care support. This resource, in the sense of 'social agency' and in the context of elder-to-elder care, means the actual capacity of older caregivers to mobilise, move and engage social networks and their members (for example family, kinship, neighbours, or informal/formal institutions; see Table 3.3) and, in so doing, expand their social space in order to generate additional material or immaterial support for older care-receivers at critical health moments. Good social relationships with children, in-laws and/or siblings are indicative of important resources for older caregivers to enhance their social agency. Gender norms, religious principles, moral values and kinship obligations as underlying cultural structures may not only limit or diminish social agency for older caregivers when mobilising additional and badly needed care support (Van Eeuwijk, 2012), but, conversely, may also strengthen and reinforce the rights, to which both older caregivers and care-receivers can lay claim, over family members and relatives.

Elder-to-elder care arrangements in Tanzania

Elder-to-elder care is not an emerging form of care support in Tanzania. But it is becoming more common due to demographic, epidemiological and social transformations in Tanzanian society over the last 20–25 years (Van Eeuwijk, 2014). Yet, both the quantity and the quality of elder-to-elder care are changing rapidly and significantly due, for example, to the out-migration of younger generations and their physical absence, the deadly impact of the HIV/AIDS epidemic on younger people, the processes of urbanisation and its concomitant change of social core units such as family and household, the new lifestyles and orientations of younger generations resulting in increasing non-compliance with care obligations to support ageing parents, the increase of economic hardships leading to restricted availability of care resources for younger providers, limited access to both formal social welfare schemes and the national health system for people growing old, the higher life expectancy resulting in an extended life span for many older people, and therefore in a distinct shift from cure to care due to older people's increasing vulnerability to non-communicable diseases and degenerative ageing impairments (see for Sub-Saharan Africa, for instance: Aboderin, 2004; Lloyd-Sherlock, 2004; Zimmer and Dayton, 2005; Van Dullemen, 2006; Velkoff and Kowal, 2006; Makoni, 2008; Whyte et al, 2008; Maher et al, 2010; HelpAge International, 2012; Alli and Maharaj, 2013; Aboderin and Beard, 2014). Elder-to-elder care is thus driven and shaped by a heterogeneity of transformative societal dynamics, representing in most cases a combination of two or more such circumstances.

Notable facets of the particular relationship 'older caregivers–older care-receivers' are reflected in the compositions of care arrangements, where exclusively older people act as both major carers and care recipients (see Table 3.1). This dimension represents the scope of social care space and distance, as well as that of gendered engagement in elder-to-elder care.

This study sample comprises 151 households where 43 older caregivers provide major care for aged people (28.5 per cent). Thus, in nearly one out of three households, primary care work for an old frail person is provided by an older woman or man. The study shows a much higher number in rural Rufiji than in highly urban Dar es Salaam, where many households have only one single older person (60 years and older), providing care for the younger children (Gerold, 2012; Simon, 2012; Van Eeuwijk, 2014; see also Obrist, Chapter Four).

Intragenerational care relations – that is, caring for members of the same generation – are strongly marked by a 'caregiving wife–care-receiving husband' dyad (see Table 3.1). This spouse relationship is indisputably the most convenient type of care arrangement among two adult people (see also Freeman, Chapter Five), as it complies with normative cultural expectations regarding care duties related to wife–husband roles. The *Warufiji* expect an aged wife to provide the best possible service to her older husband, who is entitled thereto. The following two examples reflect this perspective:

> Bibi Hadija (65) lives with her very frail husband (65) in Ikwiriri. She does all the daily household chores alone, such as cooking, washing, cleaning the house, doing the laundry, fetching water, and going to the market, but she never complains. Her son helps her occasionally by carrying a bucket of water on his bicycle; he also goes to the farm. Bibi Hadija has to do all the household work for her husband including increasingly practices of care like bathing him, accompanying him to the toilet, and buying medicine. Fortunately, her son and some of her neighbours are ready to support Bibi Hadija in times of scarcity (for example with food and water).

> Bibi Habiba (61) cares for her blind husband (64) who is completely dependent on her. Two years ago they moved from rural Rufiji to Dar es Salaam, where they live in her brother-in-law's house. Their household in Mbagala is rather poor and without any comfort – a shameful situation for her. Nevertheless, she cares for her husband devotedly every day: fetching water, washing laundry, cleaning the house, taking him to the toilet, bathing him, cooking for him, guiding him to the city, and talking to him. She considers her care activities for her husband as crucial to their marriage.

Care provision by an aged husband for his equally aged wife occurs infrequently, particularly in rural Rufiji. Generally, old *Warufiji* husbands consider extensive care support (for a frail older wife) as voluntary and optional.[3] Such situations are caused mainly by children who are unwilling or unable to care for their aged mothers, or else result from failed negotiations between parents and children and children-in-law. Care provision among older siblings – in most cases widowed,

Table 3.1: Care arrangements with older people as major caregivers for elderly care-receivers in Tanzania

Caregiver/s	Care-receiver/s	Frequency of care arrangement
Intragenerational eldercare		
wife	husband	14
1st + 2nd wife	husband	3
younger sister	older sister	1
older sister	younger brother	1
sister-in-law	brother's sister	1
husband	*wife*	4
older brother	*younger brother*	1
Intergenerational eldercare		
older daughter	mother	3
older daughter-in-law	mother-in-law	1
older granddaughter	grandmother	1
mother	older daughter	2
older son	*mother*	1
older son	*father*	1
older male cousin	*father's sister*	1
Inter- and intragenerational eldercare		
wife/daughter	husband + mother	1
wife	mother-in-law + husband	1
older granddaughter + sisters-in-law	grandmother	2
mother + older daughter	daughter/sister	1
older daughter + father/husband	*mother/wife*	2
older son + mother/wife	*father/husband*	1

Source: Fieldwork of Jana Gerold, Vendelin T Simon and Peter van Eeuwijk, 2008-11, in Dar es Salaam and Rufiji District
Note: arrangements marked in italics show men's involvement in major caregiving

divorced, or unmarried older people – is not uncommon and occurs primarily among people of the same sex as the example hereinafter discussed, illustrates. In a few Muslim families in rural Rufiji, more than one elderly wife provides care for their frail older husband.

> Babu Mohamed (79) lives with his older brother Babu Masoud (82) in Bumba, a remote village in Rufiji. Babu Mohamed, whose wife has left him, is visually impaired, cannot walk far or work any longer, and has developed Parkinson's disease. The brothers talk and chat a lot together. The older brother makes fire and looks after his younger brother when he suffers from pains. Babu Masoud organises the daily cooking, done by the younger brother's children, and the provision of water and firewood by the grandchildren. Babu Mohamed earns some money by selling tobacco and also buys food for the joint household. Babu Masoud socialises a lot with his younger brother, consoles him, and provides advice in difficult times.

Intergenerational eldercare arrangements are much less frequent due to the natural boundary of life with regard to the care-receiver. In most cases, it is an elderly daughter (60 and older) who cares for her very old mother (see Table 3.1). We found this care arrangement mostly among same-sex family members.

> Three years ago, Bibi Halima (87) moved to her elderly daughter's house in Ikwiriri. Bibi Halima lived alone for years after her husband died; gradually she felt frail and without strength and could no longer go to the farm and fetch water. Her daughter (63) has also lost her husband; she provides food for the small family, fetches water, cleans the dishes, pounds and cooks the food, and generates income. The daughter goes to the farm regularly; during this time Bibi Halima's granddaughter looks after her. Bibi Halima still helps her daughter in minor household activities; she likes living with her elderly widowed daughter.

The perception exists that care provided by older children-in-law (predominantly daughters-in-law) leads to conflicts, and is thus not wholly approved of by core kin members. Exceptions to intergenerational eldercare include aged granddaughters supporting very old grandmothers, or aged mothers caring for frail elderly daughters.

Situations combining inter- and intragenerational eldercare usually involve a very old spouse and an already elderly child (60 and older), both providing care for their very elderly mother or father (see Table 3.1). Occasionally an elderly wife (who is also a daughter) cares for her elderly husband as well as her even older mother; or two older people (for example an elderly daughter and her very aged father) provide care, respectively, for their frail elderly mother and wife.

This compilation of eldercare arrangements shows a distinct gender differentiation (see, in Table 3.1, the italicised items for men's involvement in caregiving). The vast majority of care relations presented show elderly women as the major caregivers: many more older females care for elderly men and for older women than the other way around. The aforementioned care arrangements occur mainly among close relatives due to the intimate and sensitive nature of care practices, which limits both the variety and the scope of social space.

Main care activities in elder-to-elder care arrangements and care burdens

The main care activities provided by older people for elderly people (see Table 3.2) can be grouped into three major categories:

- daily domestic work (A–H in Table 3.2);
- activities related to frailty and illness (I–M);
- emotional counselling (N–Q).

Financial issues and monetary matters were never mentioned within the scope of these care activities.

The performance of many physical domestic activities (including farm work for procuring food) is mainly due to the rural nature of our study sites in Rufiji District, where older caregivers are often still engaged in basic domestic work, such as fetching water, collecting firewood, or pounding grain (see Table 3.2). For older carers this work demands a sound physical and mental constitution. Furthermore, these many daily routine activities inside and outside the house require daily schedules that ensure that the needs of older care-receivers are not neglected.[4]

Health-related activities encompass actions inside the house (see Table 3.2: I–M). These practices centre on watching over a frail and sick elderly person, accompanying him or her to the bathroom, toilet,

Table 3.2: Main activities of care provided by elderly caregivers for aged care-receivers in Tanzania

Categories of care	Main care activities
Daily domestic work	
A	Cooking and preparation of food and drink
B	Fetching water (from outside the house)
C	Bringing water to the bathroom
D	Collecting firewood
E	Doing laundry
F	Cleaning the house/compound
G	Pounding grain
H	Going to shamba (field plot) and fetching field products, doing farm work
Activities related to frailty and illness	
I	Watching over an ill older person (when bedridden)
J	Providing food and drink
K	Accompanying to the toilet/bathroom
L	Buying medicine
M	Accompanying to hospital or to the healer
Emotional counselling	
N	Talking, gossiping, and socialising
O	Consoling and encouraging
P	Giving advice
Q	Praying together

Source: Fieldwork of Jana Gerold, Vendelin T Simon and Peter van Eeuwijk, 2008-11, in Dar es Salaam and Rufiji District

or bed and administering pharmaceuticals and healthy food, possibly a particular diet. Very intimate activities such as dressing/undressing and bathing are only provided when an older person becomes physically and mentally dependent on his or her carer(s). Only very close kin members carry out these sensitive chores. They are strongly shaped by gender roles (for instance, an older daughter cannot wash or clean the body of her frail father or dress and undress him).

Activities such as emotional counselling tend to be overlooked in most care studies. Old caregivers provide very important psychological and emotional support, as well as social assistance to elderly people in their households (see Table 3.2: N–Q). Mutually long-standing shared and even similar life experiences as well as comparable opinions make the older caregiver a trustworthy, reliable and sympathetic counsellor in a difficult situation. Talking, socialising, but also consoling, comforting, encouraging and praying together are very meaningful care activities that maintain and strengthen the emotional state of someone who is old, frail and ailing (see Obrist, Chapter Four).[5]

The great majority of elderly carers are willing and able to provide even intensive, stressful, and exhausting care for their frail aged kin – some out of free will, others out of pure necessity. Most elderly caregivers emphasised that they were not at all prepared to act as main care providers for their families in old age. Yet, their support is limited in terms of both quantity and quality. Older caregivers in the Tanzanian study sites generally identified the following four interrelated care burdens:

- physical burden;
- economic burden;
- social burden;
- emotional burden.

Older female caregivers, in particular, expect more substantial and continuous support from their family members in actively mitigating their care burdens. Instead of providing help, it is indeed the family who in many cases exerts pressure and generates unease towards elderly carers, not least by spreading rumours about 'bad care' that tarnish the social and moral reputations of aged carers. This high burden of care provision and the unmet demand for assistance can strain, even rupture, kin relations, resulting in a 'de-kinning by care'. The core understanding of the family as a reliable social 'care space', in the sense of a 'safe haven' for all of its members, is not only a highly questionable and precarious value for aged care-receivers but also for elderly caregivers who bear different and multiple care burdens in a contentious atmosphere. In the long run, such difficult circumstances have a considerable impact on the vulnerability of older caregivers – and therefore also on the vulnerability of their elderly care-receivers.

Extended care arrangements in critical health situations

In critical or problematic health situations an older caregiver may realise that his or her aged care-receiver has fallen seriously ill or is progressively weakening – and that sweeping changes at the household level are about to alter the lives of the older carer, the elderly care-receiver and their families (see also Obrist, Chapter Four). Critical health moments can be triggered by specific problematic health events which may include not only a sudden illness incident (for example, bone fracture, severe pneumonia, rapidly advancing kidney or liver disorder), which demands an immediate and adequate response, but also slow, degenerative processes that last for months and years and are monitored by the elderly caregiver and other family members. These may refer to increasing visual and auditory impairments, inguinal hernia, progressive diabetes, serious dementia, malign neoplasm and heart attacks (Van Eeuwijk, 2011; Gerold, 2012; Simon, 2012). One important agentic practice includes the social extension of an existing, but currently overstrained elder-to-elder care arrangement: new members are mobilised and 'recruited' by the older caregiver and become part (physically, financially, materially and/or emotionally) of the given care arrangement. This ability (or failure) of older caregivers to motivate and thus involve members of visible and invisible social networks (family, wider kinship or neighbourhood) to participate in care provision stands for their social agency and resilience in such serious care situations.

Table 3.3: Extended care arrangements in critical health situations in Tanzania (in households with a major older caregiver)

Main caregiver	Care receiver	Providers of additional care support
wife	husband	2nd/3rd wife
wife	husband	all children
wife	husband	son
wife	husband	daughter
wife	husband	children + son-in-law
wife	husband	son + daughter + grandchildren
wife	husband	her brother
wife	husband	neighbours
wife	husband	house tenants
older daughter	mother	grandson
older sister	older brother	grandson
younger sister	older sister	children + grandchildren (of younger sister)
husband	wife	daughter + nephew
husband	wife	her sisters
older son	mother	grandson
older son	father	daughter-in-law

Source: Fieldwork of Jana Gerold, Vendelin T Simon and Peter van Eeuwijk, 2008-11, in Dar es Salaam and Rufiji District

Table 3.3 reveals that in most care arrangement extensions children, grandchildren, children-in-law, and siblings join the existing 'older caregiver–older care-receiver' relationship. Only rarely do non-kin people become additional caregivers, for example house tenants or neighbours. Once again, close relatives are the main caregivers who join (see also Freeman, Chapter Five). Given this fact, children, grandchildren, and children-in-law are the family members who most frequently lend support to older wives in cases of problematic health situations (see Table 3.3). A gendered perspective shows that numerous men (for instance, sons, grandsons, sons-in-law and brothers) are mobilised to support the household when trying to cope with a suffering older person. In all three study sites in Tanzania the younger male and female carers who join the care-arrangement mainly contribute three care activities:

- financial support (for example buying food, paying for treatment);[6]
- physical support (for example cleaning floors, doing kitchen work);
- social support (for example socialising, consoling, giving advice).

The following two cases exemplify these extensions of social space:

> Bibi Amina (75) and her husband (85) are tenants in a small house in Mbagala. Bibi Amina could no longer provide daily care for her frail husband after it became difficult for her, due to general physical weakness, to walk unaided, even to the washroom and toilet. Finally, Bibi Amina asked their children (a son and a daughter with families) and grandchildren living only two streets away to come in and provide daily support. Besides cooking daily in their parents' house, they fetch water and wash clothes; they also provide financial assistance and socialise every day with their old parents who have become totally dependent on this kind of care support.

> Bibi Zainabu, a widow of 85 years in Ikwiriri, used to be cared for by her younger sister (82), herself an elderly widow. Bibi Zainabu has now become very weak and suffers from continuous dizziness and recurrent body pains; she can no longer leave the house and stays in her room. When her sister was no longer able to provide adequate intensive daily care for Bibi Zainabu, she begged her children and grandchildren (who live nearby) to come in and do the

daily chores, such as cooking, washing, cleaning the house, fetching water and firewood and buying food and medicine. Bibi Zainabu's brother, her cousin's children, other relatives and friends also now pay her regular visits, occasionally bringing along some money and food.

The *Warufiji* patrilineal descent system mainly arranges and adjusts care obligations in a normative way and thus limits options for alternative care settings: sons and daughters are called upon first and foremost to provide additional care for their elderly parents. Grandchildren may join these new care arrangements (see also De Klerk, Chapter Six). Marrying a younger, healthy, second or third wife is a viable response to the high burden of care experienced by the first and oldest wife, but it is not a popular option in *Warufiji* communities.

Non-kin care and institutionalised eldercare

Aged non-kin carers such as house tenants and neighbours are present in all three Tanzanian study sites (see Table 3.1 and Table 3.3), but they are not formally remunerated (see also Obrist, Chapter Four). This chapter further sheds light on another under-researched issue in Tanzania, namely formal and informal institutions where older people provide care support for other elderly, mostly frail, individuals. In almost all studied cases the chairperson, director, or principal is also an older woman or man – a fact that has an immediate, positive impact in terms of credibility, solidarity and cohesion between elderly providers (or managers) and older users/recipients (clients, members or participants).

This study has identified the following (in)formal institutions, chaired and managed by older people, whose members or participants are also older people, and whose major task is to provide care and support for aged people:

- Clubs: older men, for instance, founded an 'older male club' with informal membership, gathering regularly at the town market to sell dried tobacco. Besides providing mutual support in critical moments, they enjoy socialising and conversation with three to four older men overseeing the club's informal 'management' (case from Rufiji).
- Associations: pioneered by church institutions, government departments, or better-off older individuals. These informal 'associations of seniors', run by older leaders, undertake income-generating activities (for example chicken breeding, revolving funds), leisure time activities, religious services, home visits for social and

emotional support, and financial assistance for the ill (cases from Rufiji and Dar es Salaam).

- Self-help groups: older 'activists' founded self-help groups (for example with/for older widows and widowers who are caring for their orphaned grandchildren) with income-generating activities (for instance, making small handicrafts) and regular meetings for socialising and exchange; they enjoy occasional donations from abroad for their projects (cases from Dar es Salaam and Arusha).
- Non-governmental organisations: a couple of older men and women manage an official non-governmental organisation with funds and material donations provided by sponsors from abroad; they visit their older frail clients at home on a daily basis, which includes administering drugs, or they run an office providing legal assistance to elderly people (cases from Dar es Salaam, Arusha and Moshi).
- Formal care institutions: an old people's or nursing home run by faith-based organisations (for example a Catholic order of nuns) or typically managed by older people, for elderly residents who reside there on a permanent basis (cases from Dar es Salaam and Zanzibar).

Care work in the above-mentioned institutions is mainly carried out by older women and without remuneration (except for formal care institutions and in part for non-governmental organisations). In such institutions Christian charity, professional ethics of service, past personal experience, a sense of belonging along with feelings of solidarity among people of the same age (and sex), and activism triggered by notions of gender or age inequality appear as the main reasons and motivations for providing care support to older people. For elderly people in acute or long-term need of care, these institutions and their aged principals play an increasingly crucial role due to their complementary nature in terms of social, emotional, economic and health support (see Obrist, Chapter Four; De Klerk, Chapter Six; Van der Geest, Chapter One; Hoffman, Chapter Seven; and Pype, Chapter Two). They represent an active part of non-kin 'community support' by expanding the 'social space of care' (including care practices) for both caregivers and care-receivers, but without transgressing the normative boundaries of eldercare. However, they cannot fully replace family and kin as core and intimate care providers in Tanzania.

A number of older caregivers in these (in)formal institutions have developed valuable 'soft skills' such as fundraising, proposal writing, public relations skills and worldwide networking through new social media.[7] Their initiatives aim not least at the global 'care market', where care activities targeting older frail people in Sub-Saharan Africa sell increasingly well. Tanzania's late 1970s and 1980s modernist development era brought new ideas, actors and technologies, as well as the rationality of 'modern' project and programme management. Some previously mentioned care-providing institutions (particularly the last four) have turned into formal and informal 'care projects' or 'health programmes', funded and supported by national and international private or public donors.[8] 'Project course instruments', such as planning, monitoring, evaluation and accountability, represent new values in care work for local older caregivers as managers or directors of such institutions. The formalisation of such care work transforms non-kin eldercare into a commodity ('care labour') within such 'carescapes' (also see Obrist, Chapter Four). At the same time they form entry-points for new, flexible and thus rapidly changing, scientific, political and lay concepts concerning ageing, health and care practices. On the one hand, these inter-institutional and transnational connections, and the inherent production, exchange and transfer of concepts, ideas, images and imaginations, and experiences on care work shape and challenge new forms of inter- and intragenerational care relations at the local level. On the other hand, a different old-age vulnerability results from these eldercare institutions: an increasing dependence on project funding and foreign donors creates new forms of vulnerability for the older caregivers and aged care-receivers who must now rely on these eldercare institutions.

Discussion

The quality and quantity of care provided by elderly people for older people in their households is widely underestimated and often simply overlooked. Two main reasons for this attitude emerge from this research: first, elder-to-elder care does not comply with social norms and cultural rules; it therefore does not conform to the 'right' practice of care relation and fails to comply with conventional images of eldercare. In other words, it does not occupy the 'right' social space of care provision. Second, older caregivers themselves display an increased degree of multiple vulnerabilities and are considered to be less resilient and therefore not 'ideal' providers of appropriate 'good' care. In all three settings of this study – rural and urban, patrilineal, Muslim *Warufiji* – normative discourses on intergenerational relations, care support and kinship obligations are notable for the high expectations of old people in need of care, who state that their children must provide care (Van Eeuwijk, 2011; 2014; Simon, 2012). This image and imagination are distinct expressions of complying with normative cultural requirements of filial piety and kinship obligations, thus limiting the scope of social space with regard to eldercare.

This ideal view of intergenerational indebtedness does not tally with real care arrangements: in about one third of the study's households an older person provides major care for another aged individual (60 and older). Strictly speaking, one could argue that intergenerational relations and parent–child negotiations have completely failed in these families as also has, implicitly, the notion of the family as central care provider. Nevertheless, everyday practice shows that explicit social blame is neither placed on elder (caring) parents nor on their (non-caring) children.[9] In our Tanzanian study communities older caregivers judge this elder-to-elder care arrangement to be a necessary but also pragmatic adjustment to a rapidly changing urban and rural context, even as they tacitly miss the much praised sense of intergenerational reciprocity. In Tanzania older caregivers regard this care arrangement as an unfortunate situation that must be accepted under the circumstances – but implicitly it goes against social conventions and transgresses established norms of care. This 'idealized morality' (Utomo, 2002, 226),[10] according to which care support from children is desired, has partially failed; it does not, however, undermine the lived organisation of moral norms, social structures and religious values. In fact, high levels of assistance from younger children is no longer expected – except in problematic health circumstances – and new practices of elder-to-elder care are becoming increasingly well established.

Two interacting fields shape this elder-to-elder care in Tanzania: cultural and social structures represented by norms, rules, conventions and values (for example, filial piety, kinship obligations, gender relations, religious standards,[11] moral principles, and underlying social imagery) frame ageing and care relations in very normative ways; and social agency enables older carers to mediate practice options, enhancing their capacity to act, for instance, through negotiation, refusal and divorce (see Van der Geest, Chapter One), and by extending care arrangements, using urban–rural resources, converting social capital into 'actions', involving (in)formal eldercare institutions and using technologies (for example, mobile phones). Yet, some agentic practices, such as an elderly wife's strict refusal to provide care, go against conventions of care provision and lead to harsh reactions. The most frequent intragenerational form of eldercare in Tanzania, namely when an elderly wife cares for her aged husband, essentially complies with prevailing gender norms – even though it is not an intergenerational care arrangement and thus not considered ideal (Van Eeuwijk, 2014). Moreover, in times of critical health circumstances, these new joint care arrangements draw upon well-accepted conventions such as kinship obligations, children's indebtedness and intergenerational support, thus fully complying with cultural imaginations of 'good' care.

The multiple burdens of older carers increase their degree of vulnerability, and thus, as we argue, the degree of vulnerability of their aged care-receivers. Nonetheless, these cases show that older caregivers responsible for aged care-receivers going through critical health incidents usually make the most of their social and cultural capital. They are able to diminish their own degree of vulnerability, and thus the vulnerability of their charges through, for instance, mobilising younger kin members to participate in care work and join new 'combined' inter- and intragenerational care arrangements. These 'changing webs of kinship' (Alber et al, 2010, 43) or extensions of 'social care space' have both weaknesses and strengths. The case of the patrilineal *Warufiji* shows a rather restricted optionality for creating new extended care arrangements, and the prospect of expanding social spaces for care matters in critical health moments is somewhat restricted by norms, rules and values. In contrast, these same restrictive rules and values in *Warufiji* communities entitle an older woman or man in need of care to claim effective support from his or her spouse, children and younger siblings: this is an important reassurance as well as a final means of putting pressure on family and kin. Where these members do not respond to such claims, elder-to-elder care arrangements become reality – against convention, but accepted!

Tanzania's many informal, as well as a few formal institutions providing care for older people, in particular those social bodies where older people care for other older people who are frail, mainly provide complementary care support for older people in need. In a few cases they act as a last (care) resort for socially excluded and economically neglected elderly people. Common indicators of institutional identification, such as same age, religion, sex, marital status, locality, illness or care burden, as well as peer 'management', undoubtedly lead to a high degree of credibility and reliability from an elderly care-receiver's perspective (see also Hoffman, Chapter Seven). The expansion of many of these (in)formal elder-to-elder care institutions into projects and programmes of 'global health' – thus following their own developmental rationalities – increasingly turns these institutions into not only meaningful links in global care chains, but also into important non-kin 'partners' for families and households when social spaces of care have to be expanded at problematic health moments. They become active 'gatekeepers' for the transfer of new care practice models and images. Moreover, through the local appropriation of transcultural flows, these elder-to-elder care institutions, as globally linked projects, act as 'new' social spaces and places of care, and as vital innovative platforms – in the sense of 'carescapes' developing some form of shared care citizenship and care-based sociality among older caregivers and care-receivers – and thus have an increasing impact on old-age vulnerability in Tanzania.

Notes

[1] See Acknowledgements.

[2] The percentage of the total population aged 60 years and older in Tanzania was 4.9 per cent in 2012; life expectancy at birth (2012–15) reaches 58 years for men and 60 years for women in Tanzania (HelpAge International, 2012).

[3] *Warufiji* gender norms stipulate that an older husband is obliged to provide financial support and allocate required household resources for his wife. But in actual fact husbands provide more 'invisible' care support than clearly visible and tangible relief.

[4] Important markers in the daily routines of care-dependent older people are meals and commensality (see Van Eeuwijk, 2007). At the same time, these routine care activities may exert considerable control and power over older care-receivers (Van Eeuwijk, 2007).

[5] Mobile phones play an important role in personal counselling and emotional support for older people in all three study areas (see Gerold (2011; 2012) and Simon (2012)).

[6] This includes remittances (for instance, from children working in other cities in Tanzania or even abroad [mainly in the Gulf States and the USA]), bank orders sent through mobile phones and cash money that passes through a third party (for example, a bus driver, neighbour or close friend). These modes of cash transfer for older parents are well established in the small rural town of Ikwiriri (Rufiji District), a regional out-migration centre that acts as hub in a longer step–migration chain (see also Obrist (Tanzania), Van der Geest (Ghana) and Hoffman (South Africa) – Chapters Four, One and Seven, respectively).

[7] Prince (2014, 79) has emphasised the acquired (biomedical) knowledge of HIV-positive Kenyans in non-governmental organisations, which provides self-empowerment and strengthens the feeling of becoming a subject of development.

[8] See the interesting approach of 'projectification' in the HIV/AIDS field (in Uganda) developed by Meinert and Whyte (2014): not only are many new AIDS projects in the health care system founded, but anti-retroviral treatment patients also become

'clients' in health care projects (for instance, having an electronic file, a research study number and a personal counsellor).

[9] In all three study areas – and in urban Dar es Salaam in particular – older people state that nowadays older as well as younger people face enough difficulties to make ends meet, and that this is why many older people refrain from urging younger people to provide care for them at all costs (see also Hoffman and De Klerk – Chapters Seven and Six, respectively).

[10] Utomo (2002, 226) has studied the sexual values and experiences of young unmarried urban Indonesians and refers to 'an "idealized morality" fuelled by religious norms and teachings, and traditional social values [that] still exists…and still has a strong influence on the young and old generation'. New values are adopted, but they must not endanger this 'idealised morality' and thus undermine the moral order and authority.

[11] The Qur'an provides some commanding guidance regarding filial piety and intergenerational obligation, for instance, in Surah 17: 23–4 ('[A]nd, kindness to your parents, whether one or both of them attain old age with thee: and say not to them, "Fie!" neither reproach them; but speak to them both with respectful speech; And defer humbly to them out of tenderness') and Surah 31: 14 ('We have commanded man concerning his parents. His mother carrieth him with weakness upon weakness; nor until after two years is he weaned. Be grateful to me, and to thy parents. Unto me shall all come') (Margoliouth and Rodwell, 2012, 131, 200).

Acknowledgements

The author wishes to thank Nigel Stephenson and Isabelle de Rezende for their English proofreading and the reviewers for their valuable and helpful comments.

This research project in Tanzania ('From "Cure to Care" among the Elderly. Old-age Vulnerability in Tanzania', 2008–11; head: Peter van Eeuwijk) was funded by the Swiss National Science Foundation (SNSF). This institution is also funding the current research project in Tanzania ('Ageing, Agency and Health in Urbanizing Tanzania', 2012–15; head: Brigit Obrist; major research sites: Dar es Salaam and Zanzibar; minor research sites: Arusha and Moshi), from where some first findings have also been considered in this chapter. Jana Gerold, Vendelin T Simon, Andrea Grolimund, Sandra Staudacher and Tanzanian field assistants collected the empirical data together with the project heads.

References

Aboderin, I, 2004, Modernisation and ageing theory revisited: Current explanations of recent developing world and historical western shifts in material family support for older people, *Ageing and Society* 24, 29–50

Aboderin, I, Beard, JR, 2014, Older people's health in sub-Saharan Africa, *The Lancet* 385, e9–e11

Alber, E, Häberlein, T, Jeannett, M, 2010, Changing webs of kinship: Spotlights on West Africa, *Africa Spectrum* 3, 43–67

Alli, F, Maharaj, P, 2013, The health situation of older people in Africa, in P Maharaj (ed) *Aging and health in Africa*, pp 53–89, New York: Springer, International Perspectives on Aging 4

Ardington, C, Case, A, Islam, M, Lam, D, Leibbrandt, M, Menendez, A, Olgiati, A, 2010, The impact of AIDS on intergenerational support in South Africa: Evidence from the Cape area panel study, *Research on Aging* 32, 1, 97–121

Bongaarts, J, Zimmer, Z, 2002, Living arrangements of older adults in the developing world: An analysis of demographic and health survey household surveys, *Journal of Gerontology* 57B, 3, S145–57

EveryChild and HelpAge International, 2012, Family first: Prioritising support to kinship carers, especially older carers, *Working Paper* 4, London: EveryChild UK

Gerold, J, 2011, Kommunizieren ohne Worte: Wie ältere Menschen in Tansania Mobiltelefone benutzen, *Afrika-Bulletin* 142, 6–7

Gerold, J, 2012, Full of life: Old age and care in urban Dar es Salaam, Tanzania, Unpublished PhD Dissertation, Basel: University of Basel

Gerold, J, 2013, On the move: Elderly people living the city of Dar es Salaam, Tanzania, in B Obrist, V Arlt, E Macamo (eds) *Living the city in Africa: Processes of invention and intervention*, pp 153–70, Münster: LIT Verlag

HelpAge International, 2004, *The cost of love: Older people in the fight against AIDS in Tanzania*, London: HelpAge International

HelpAge International, 2012, *Ageing in the twenty-first century: A celebration and a challenge*, London: HelpAge International

Kleinman, A, 2009, Caregiving: The odyssey of becoming more human, *The Lancet* 373, 292–3

Kleinman, A, Van der Geest, S, 2009, 'Care' in health care: Remaking the moral world of medicine, *Medische Antropologie* 21, 159–68

De Klerk, J, 2011, *Being old in times of AIDS: Aging, caring and relating in Northwest Tanzania*, Leiden: Africa Studies Centre

Lloyd-Sherlock, P, 2004, Ageing, development and social protection: Generalisations, myths and stereotypes, in P Lloyd-Sherlock (ed) *Living longer: Ageing, development and social protection*, pp 1–17, London: Zed Books

Maher, D, Smeeth, L, Sekajugo, J, 2010, Health transition in Africa: Practical policy proposals for primary care, *Bulletin of the World Health Organization* 88, 943–8

Makoni, S, 2008, Aging in Africa: A critical review, *Journal of Cross-Cultural Gerontology* 23, 199–209

Margoliouth, G, Rodwell, JM (trans), 2012, *The Koran by Mohammed*, Lawrence, KS: Digireads.com Publishing

Meinert, L, Whyte, SR, 2014, Epidemic projectification: AIDS responses in Uganda as event and process, *Cambridge Anthropology* 32, 1, 77–94

Ministry of Labour, Youth Development and Sports, 2003, *National ageing policy United Republic of Tanzania*, Dar es Salaam: Ministry of Labour, Youth Development and Sports

Mol, A, Moser, I, Pols, J, 2010, Care: Putting practice into theory, in A Mol, I Moser, J Pols (eds) *Care in practice: On tinkering in clinics, homes and farms*, pp 7–25, Bielefeld: Transcript

Ogunmefun, C, Gilbert, L, Schatz, E, 2011, Older female caregivers and HIV/AIDS-related secondary stigma in rural South Africa, *Journal of Cross-Cultural Gerontology* 26, 1, 85–102

Prince, RJ, 2014, Precarious projects: Conversions of (biomedical) knowledge in an East African city, *Medical Anthropology* 33, 1, 68–83

Schnegg, M, Pauli, J, Beer, B, Alber, E, 2010, Verwandtschaft heute: Positionen, Ergebnisse und Forschungsperspektiven, in E Alber, B Beer, J Pauli, M Schnegg (eds) *Verwandtschaft heute: Positionen, Ergebnisse und Perspektiven*, pp 7–44, Berlin: Dietrich Reimer Verlag

Simon, VT, 2012, *Ageing, health and care in rural Tanzania*, Unpublished PhD Dissertation, Basel: University of Basel

Sokolovsky, J, 2009, A global vision of aging, culture and context, in J Sokolovsky (ed) *The cultural context of aging: Worldwide perspectives*, pp 1–12, Westport, CT: Praeger

Ssengonzi, R, 2009, The impact of HIV/AIDS on the living arrangements and well-being of elderly caregivers in rural Uganda, *AIDS Care* 21, 3, 309–14

Tronto, JC, 2009, *Moral boundaries: A political argument for an ethic of care*, New York: Routledge

Utomo, ID, 2002, Sexual values and early experiences among young people in Jakarta, in L Manderson, P Liamputtong (eds) *Coming of age in South and Southeast Asia: Youth, courtship and sexuality*, pp 207–27, Richmond, VA: Curzon

Van Dullemen, C, 2006, Older people in Africa: New engines to society?, *National Women's Studies Association (NWSA) Journal* 18, 99–105

Van Eeuwijk, P, 2006a, Altern im städtischen Umfeld Indonesiens, in P van Eeuwijk, B Obrist (eds) *Vulnerabilität, Migration und Altern: Medizinethnologische Ansätze im Spannungsfeld von Theorie und Praxis*, pp 218–40, Zürich: Seismo Verlag

Van Eeuwijk, P, 2006b, Old-age vulnerability, ill-health and care support in urban areas of Indonesia, *Ageing and Society* 26, 61–80

Van Eeuwijk, P, 2007, The power of food: Mediating social relationships in the care of chronically ill elderly people in urban Indonesia, *Anthropology of Food* S3, 1–23

Van Eeuwijk, P, 2011, Altern in Unsicherheit: Gesundheit und Pflege von alten Menschen in Indonesien und Tansania, in C Kollewe, E Schenkel (eds) *Alter: unbekannt. Über die Vielfalt des Älterwerdens. Internationale Perspektiven*, pp 83–111, Bielefeld: Transcript Verlag

Van Eeuwijk, P, 2012, Pains, pills, and physicians: Self-medication as social agency among elderly people in urban Sulawesi, Indonesia, in B Röder, W de Jong, KW Alt (eds) *Alter(n) anders denken: Kulturelle und biologische Perspektiven*, pp 257–79, Köln: Böhlau Verlag, Kulturgeschichte der Medizin 2

Van Eeuwijk, P, 2014, The elderly providing care for the elderly in Tanzania and Indonesia: Making 'elder-to-elder' care visible, *Sociologus* 64, 1, 29–52

Velkoff, VA, Kowal, PR, 2006, Aging in sub-Saharan Africa: The changing demography of the region, in B Cohen, J Menken (eds) *Aging in sub-Saharan Africa: Recommendations for furthering research*, pp 55–91, Washington, DC: The National Academies Press

Whyte, SR, Alber, E, Van der Geest, S, 2008, Generational connections and conflicts in Africa: An introduction, in E Alber, S van der Geest, SR Whyte (eds) *Generations in Africa: Connections and conflicts*, pp 1–23, Münster: LIT Verlag

WHO (World Health Organization), 2002, *Impact of AIDS on older people in Africa: Zimbabwe case study*, Geneva: WHO

Zimmer, Z, Dayton, J, 2005, Older adults in sub-Saharan Africa living with children and grandchildren, *Population Studies* 59, 3, 295–312

FOUR

Place matters: the home as a key site of old-age care in coastal Tanzania

Brigit Obrist

Introduction

> When I was young, I was a farmer in Ikwiriri. Every day I walked long distances to my fields in the river valley. Then I moved and settled in Dar es Salaam. But as I grew older, I slowly started being unable to walk long distances with my goods in my hands. I decided to close my business; I came back to the village, and then completely moved to the fields for the entire agricultural season. I could no longer manage to walk every day [from the village to the farm and back again]. This situation was made worse by illness; I developed a painful *busha*.[1] My scrotum swelled up and grew bigger and bigger. Finally I could not walk anymore, and stopped walking and working entirely. See, this is ageing! It started slowly! Slowly! Until it pinned me down!

The story of the 78-year-old Mzee[2] Hafith vividly illustrates that place becomes increasingly important in older age. As a young man, he first worked as a farmer, moving easily between the village and the floodplains where he cultivated rice and other food crops. He then migrated to the city and became a petty trader, walking the streets and peddling his merchandise. As he grew older and weaker, carrying weights and walking far became increasingly troublesome. He returned to the village and his rice fields, until an advanced stage of his illness made him stop walking and working. Ageing gradually 'pinned him down'.

This chapter asks what happens when older people like Mzee Hafith become restricted in their movements. What spaces of care become significant, or even open up, while others close down? Grounded in empirical research, it suggests a theoretically informed approach paying particular attention to the spatial[3] dimensions of older people's ageing and care experiences.

Because the experience of ageing is intricately linked with the body, I use an embodiment perspective as a starting point for my inquiry. In the phenomenological perspective, an ill person apprehends the body both a) 'as lived body (the body experienced at the pre-reflective level in a non-objective way)', and b) 'as objective or physiological body (the body apprehended at the reflective level as a material objective entity among other entities within the world)' (Toombs, 1993, 51). Most of the time, in our everyday lives, we are not aware of our lived body. We use our senses of seeing or hearing and carry out the daily activities of walking or working without giving it much thought. Old age, illness and disability, however, turn daily life – which before had simply happened without the need for self-awareness – into a series of events to be faced, whether due to discomfort, unease, pain or inability to perform as usual. I refer to these events as 'critical health moments'. From a methodological point of view, it is especially during these critical health moments that older people, and those with whom they interact, articulate their experiences of health and care through discursive or enacted practice. During critical health moments, we also become aware of 'lived spatiality and temporality', as Kay Toombs (2001) impressively explicates in a phenomenological description and interpretation of her own experience of multiple sclerosis. Through her narrative account, we can re-experience how the illness affected her ability to see, hear, sit and stand, and thus begin to comprehend that her lived relationship with space and time has become progressively more unsettling.

The geographer David Seamon (2014) introduces the concept of 'environmental embodiment' to refer to the ways in which our lived body experiences disruptive events and engages with space and time. Drawing on the phenomenology of Merleau-Ponty (1962), he suggests that old age, illness and disability upset 'body routines' (sets of coordinated corporal actions sustaining a specific task or aim, for example, driving or cooking) and 'time–space routines' (sets of more or less habitual bodily actions that extend through a considerable portion of time, for example a getting-up routine or a going-to-church routine).

In line with a phenomenological perspective, this study draws on the notion that 'space becomes place when it is used and lived' (Cresswell, 2004, 2). I will argue that for old, ill and disabled people, the home becomes a place of particular importance. It is important to note, though, that home 'as a species of "lived space"...appears to be an inherently ambiguous phenomenon' (Tuedio, 2009, 284). A key paradox is that 'home' can be a built structure with clear boundaries, but it can also reflect a 'field of experience' (Tuedio, 2009, 298–9). In the second sense, being at home means belonging to a 'field of interrelatedness' or a 'field of intimate involvements', which offers protection against 'uncanny assaults on our vulnerabilities' (Tuedio, 2009, 288). But despite the common assumption that the home space represents a zone of safety, comfort and security, home is often a place of ongoing contestation, where vulnerabilities and dependencies are potentially exposed (Tuedio, 2009, 285). As a lived space, the home is not enclosed and clearly demarcated, but is rather in continuous interaction with the outside world, its cultural meanings and power structures (Johansson and Saarikangas, 2009, 11).

The home, in other words, intersects with broader lived spaces of care or 'carescapes'. The suffix '–scape' indicates 'that these are not objectively given relations that look the same from every angle of vision but, rather, that they are deeply perspectival constructs, inflected by the historical, linguistic, and political situatedness of different sorts of actors' (Appadurai, 2005, 33). By introducing the term 'carescapes' the study emphasises that lived spaces of care are created at the intersections of embodied people, the home and broader society, which in turn increasingly shapes and is shaped by global connections. These places cannot be neatly separated. The intimate, every day, care of frail and disabled older people occurs at their shifting intersections.

Study sites and methodology

The study presented here is based on ethnographic research on ageing, health and care of a much broader scope (see also Van Eeuwijk, Chapter Three). Two consecutive research projects have been carried out in coastal Tanzania.[4] They started:

- in two rural sites in the Rufiji District and an urban neighbourhood in Dar es Salaam with many migrants from Rufiji (2008–11); and
- expanded to include other urban neighbourhoods of Dar es Salaam and the city of Zanzibar, as well as transnational links with the United States and Oman (2012–16).

The Rufiji District is located about 178 kilometres south of Dar es Salaam. One of the rural study sites was Ikwiriri, a centrally located cluster of villages near the floodplains, which is rapidly growing into a small town, especially since the building of the Mkapa Bridge across the Rufiji River, connecting the main road from Dar es Salaam with Lindi and Mtwara further south. The other rural study site was Bumba village, an isolated location off the main road, about 80 kilometres from Ikwiriri, and consisting of a cluster of hamlets in an elevated area far from the floodplains.

Dar es Salaam, a bustling port city on the East African Coast of the Indian Ocean, attracts many migrants from all parts of Tanzania (see Obrist, 2006). It has a population of nearly 4.5 million (NBS, 2013) and is among the fastest growing cities in Africa. Although Dar es Salaam has seen an unprecedented construction boom in the past decade, more than 80 per cent of its residents live in unplanned, unserviced areas with poor infrastructure, irregular water supply, and frequent power cuts (UN-HABITAT, 2010, 13). The project was carried out in five neighbourhoods (*mitaa*) representing urban heterogeneity: Mbagala and Kijangani in Temeke Municipality, Ilala Mafuriko in Ilala Municipality, and Manzese Mnasi Moja and Ada Estate in Kinondoni Municipality.

Zanzibar City is located on an island roughly due north of Dar es Salaam across the Zanzibar Channel. Its historical architecture reflects the diverse influences underlying Swahili culture, with a unique mixture of Arab, Persian, Indian and European elements. In 2000, the city was designated as a UNESCO World Heritage Site (Hitchcock, 2002). Today it attracts tourists from all parts of the world and has a population of about 220,000 (NBS, 2013). To capture the heterogeneity of this urban space, four neighbourhoods (*shehia*) were selected: Mpendae, Chumbuni, Kikwajuni and Shangani.

In the rural and urban research sites, the field research teams interviewed a total of 260 older people in their homes, and then carried out an extended follow-up process with a sub-sample of 110 older people, using the official definition of old age as 60+ years of age (URT, 2003). Interviews were conducted in Swahili, tape-recorded and then translated into English.

This chapter focuses on about a third of the study participants who were *sina nguvu* at the time of the first interview (n=82). The Swahili phrase *sina nguvu* ('I don't have strength') refers to a health condition marked by a series of critical moments due to old age, illness and injury, leaving the older men and women frail and no longer able to perform their gendered routines. The age of the *sina nguvu* study participants ranged from 60 to 102 years. Since it is assumed that both author and readers are used to thinking of old people in terms of chronological age, the age in years for each quoted study participant has been noted; however, it is neither relevant for the participants nor for the definition of a *sina nguvu* case. In terms of geographical distribution, the remote village of Bumba had the highest proportion of *sina nguvu* cases (42 per cent), followed by the rural town of Ikwiriri (35 per cent), Zanzibar city (24 per cent) and Dar es Salaam (22 per cent).

The body

Unsurprisingly, many narrative accounts by older people in the *sina nguvu* category report a gradual decline in strength, sometimes complicated by an illness, as illustrated by the case of Mzee Hafith from Ikwiriri at the beginning of this chapter. Mzee Juma (84 years old) who spent his whole life in and around Dar es Salaam did not suffer from a specific disease, but the common signs of old age, such as weak legs, numb hands, poor sight and too few teeth caused him to experience his body as almost an adversary. 'I have strength to work, my mind (*roho*: spirit) tells me. I would do it because I am used to farming, but my body does not want [to work], so I fail.' Still other old men suffered from diseases that gradually invaded their bodies and took control, as Mzee Mahir (97 years old) from the remote village Bumba explained:

> Do you see me? I am shaking. If I keep talking without a rest, then you might see that this part, the left part, especially the arm is as though falling off, or it looks like it wants to hit you. This is such a terrible disease; it is horrible. I tell you, I see myself dying. Every day it is getting worse; it does not improve. If I am very tired then it is like I am going to collapse at any time. Not only am I shaking, but speaking is also difficult; my chest is like full of air...It is tough and difficult. I have been to hospitals and to traditional healers. Now I have come to terms with the fact that this is the end...Last time I was in Dar...after the doctor checked my health, he told us that it is called Parkinson disease. I have my certificates. He told us that it is difficult to get treated... Since then, my condition has not gotten better. Last year we met in the school building, but this year I can't walk there anymore. When you come next year, I may not be able to come outside like this anymore, and the year after that you will only meet me in a grave. It is going so fast, and it is getting me down so quickly.

This passage illustrates how Mzee Mahir's body, mind and emotions, in fact his whole life, have become dominated by the disease. Not only does he have a disease, he is seriously ill and he knows he will die. The mind–body dualism breaks down, not just in the painful body (Jackson, 1994, 208), but also in the ageing body, especially if the person suffers from a life-threatening condition. The sensory and emotional experiences described as weakness, numbness, pain and tremor are thus not only bodily signs; they make old people constantly aware of their lived bodies, threaten their selves, and turn their everyday lives into a series of critical health moments.

In this process, the older people become increasingly aware of the spatial – and temporal – dimensions of their lived bodies. Bibi Ashura (85 years old) from Ikwiriri used visual language to recount how disease – in her case chronic diarrhoea – limited her scope of action.

> This is exactly the problem of being sick. You get cornered, and your movements are reduced. Slowly the disease hunts you, chasing you hundreds of miles while you try to escape. Finally it reduces you until it catches you in bed. Then what! Your movements are only on the bed, and still it continues hunting you until you cannot even turn anymore. You try, but it is just pain everywhere. You just lie flat and still on the bed until you die.

These quotes demonstrate how existential the body's spatial and temporal dimensions have become for older people who have lost their strength, whether they live in a remote village like Bumba, a rural town like Ikwiriri, or metropolitan centres like Dar es Salaam or Zanzibar. In their view, the body has turned into an agent that can no longer be controlled; in the end the body 'pins you down', 'puts you down', and 'blocks you from working'. 'You get cornered' and 'your movements are reduced', until you end up 'flat and still on the bed' and finally die. As one woman put it, 'the elderly body becomes a home to illness'. Such dramatic statements mirror the fact that several of the study participants had reached the end of their lives. Nine of them actually died during or shortly after our field research.

If all *sina nguvu* cases were grouped along a space–time continuum, they would range from

- still able to occasionally leave the house and engage in some activities but no longer capable of working (n=19); to
- moving only within and around the house and performing a few livelihood or domestic tasks (n=52); and
- being bedridden (n=11).

Most older people were thus in the mid-range, and found 'body routines' and 'time–space routines' (Seamon, 2014) increasingly difficult to perform. What they used to do without thinking, like getting up, standing and walking, squatting in the toilet, taking a shower, getting dressed and undressed, using their hands to grasp things, or make mats or pots, and biting and swallowing food, has now become a challenge. The men recounted that they could no longer farm, or make a living in the city, cut firewood, renovate the house, or go to the shops or the market, and that their participation in political events, prayers at the mosque and family cycle celebrations was severely curtailed. Women's accounts centred around their difficulties in pounding grain, cooking, sweeping, fetching water and carrying buckets of water to the toilet, including for their husbands; and they deplored not being able to take part in initiation rituals, weddings and burials. A frequently heard sentence was: 'Nipo tu!' (I am just here – without doing anything.)

Still, in the rural and the urban sites, older men performed duties of, for instance, house guards, while older women kept an eye on small children when their daughters were busy working. These may seem like minor activities compared to the tasks they used to fulfil when they were younger and healthier, but such small tasks kept them busy and showed that they were still able to contribute to family life. The older people themselves emphasised this point in their narratives. I thus agree with Freeman (Chapter Five) that narrating – but also performing – such small acts of self-care and reciprocity also indicates strategies for maintaining positive 'adult' identities.

The home

Many of the older people in this study talked about their homes as physical structures that they built or bought. From an outsider's perspective, the material differences among the homes were enormous and mirrored broader social and economic changes. In Bumba, most *sina nguvu* older people lived in very basic self-made shelters with outdoor washrooms and squat latrines 10 to 30 metres away from the main living spaces. In Dar es Salaam and Zanzibar, several older people stayed in crowded and poorly serviced houses, while others resided in spacious cement buildings, equipped with indoor bathrooms as well as toilet bowls and seats.

I stress the toilet and bathing facilities because these features, and the relative difficulty or ease of reaching and using them, were common topics brought up by study participants. Another feature frequently mentioned across study sites was the verandah (*baraza*). Sitting in these open spaces, watching people pass by, and having an occasional chat was a favourite pastime for many old men and women. The radio, or a television set in the better-off homes, rarely came up in their accounts but nonetheless played a role in the lives of many older people, as the home visits carried out during the follow-up studies have shown.

Considering the home as, not only a physical structure, but as a field of experience, interrelatedness and intimate involvements (Tuedio, 2009) shifts our attention to the question: who comes to the help of older people when they are no longer able to perform livelihood and domestic activities? Care arrangements were diverse, but three common configurations can be discerned:

- a person living in the home of the old person becomes the main caregiver;
- a person living elsewhere comes to help;
- the old person is moved to the home of a caregiver.

Since livelihood and domestic activities are deeply embedded in gendered and generational divisions of labour, arrangements for older men and women shall be examined separately.

The caregiver lives in the old person's home

Help for older men usually came from their wives who, in turn, were often supported by their daughters and granddaughters. We are referring once more to the example of Mzee Mahir in Bumba, but similar situations have been observed in all study sites.

> Mzee Mahir lived with his wife and daughter. Before they went out, usually to work in the fields, the women prepared his food and put it near the place where he rested. His wife often inquired how he felt and whether he needed anything special. She asked what he wanted to eat and organised his meals and his days. She did his laundry, boiled water, brought it to the bathroom and helped him with bathing. She also gave him company and represented him at community events. They discussed what was going on in the village and shared future plans. Their daughter helped her mother with common household tasks like cooking, cleaning, doing laundry, fetching water and collecting firewood. She also supported her in cultivating the family's fields, went to the village shop and fetched medicine in

Kibiti, the next bigger settlement. His wife admitted that she often felt overwhelmed by the work because their daughter could only help with housework chores and cultivation but not with the intimate care of her father.

Avoidance rules based on gender and generation restricted daughters from performing intimate care tasks for their fathers, such as washing their bed sheets, underpants or bodies. These tasks were carried out by the wives who sometimes also gave massages to relieve back and leg pains. Several old men became so dependent that they felt neglected if their wife spent a few days in the fields or visiting relatives, even if they lived in a large extended household. Clearly the rules left spaces for expectations, interpretations and contestations among those involved in care relationships; we, however, did not systematically record them as, for example, De Klerk (Chapter Six), Hoffman (Chapter Seven) and Van der Geest (Chapter One) have done (in this volume).

As the example of Mzee Mahir's wife indicates, the double burden of everyday routines and special care activities for a dependent husband could become onerous for older women (see also Chapter Three by Van Eeuwijk). It was quite common for an older man to marry and live with a much younger wife, especially if the older wife had died, been divorced, or left him to move back to her own kin. Such disruptions were often painful and involved not only the older couple but also their closest kin. In such cases, the home became a site of tensions and conflict among genders and generations (Johansson and Saarikangas, 2009, 17). Moreover, there was no guarantee that a young wife would provide good care. Two old men in Dar es Salaam ended up taking care of their much younger wives because they fell seriously ill, and similar stories have been recorded in the rural areas.

For older women, help usually came from a daughter and/or grandchildren, and in a few cases from a sister or a sister-in-law. Some better-off women in the urban areas had a paid housemaid (*dada*), like Bibi Sharifa, 80 years old, from Zanzibar who lived with her daughter in her late husband's house.

> I can't do any kitchen activities. I can't do them anymore, but the children are doing them for me. I rarely stay in the kitchen. Laundry and many other activities, I cannot do anymore. *Dada* cleans the dishes. If I try to clean the dishes I feel numbness (*ganzi*). Even to sweep the floor I have to call somebody to help. Or when I have finished eating, I call someone. I cannot lift heavy things. But I can still

walk to the toilet and back. Yes, I can. Sometimes, when I feel that my body is heavy, the children will ask *dada* to prepare warm water and put it in the bathroom. I can't take a shower, they have to help me.

For old mothers who were confined to a room, daughters usually organised care around the bed, as the example of Bibi Aisha, 98 years, from Ikwiriri illustrates.

Bibi Aisha stayed inside the house and could not walk anymore. Her daughter prepared her meals and put the plate and spoon on the chair near her bed. Bibi Aisha struggled to move over to the toilet and the bathing facility placed beside her bed. She used a cup for bathing while sitting on a chair; sometimes she had to be helped. Bibi Aisha did not want to be taken to the hospital anymore; she thought her time had come. She actually passed away during field research.

Since her daughter was busy earning a living by cultivating food crops, this old woman was left alone during the day. When possible, daughters arranged for grandchildren or other relatives to look after bedridden patients when they had to leave the homestead.

The caregiver comes to the old person's home

A few old men in Ikwiriri and Dar es Salaam lived alone and received meals and some domestic help from sisters and daughters who had their own homes.

Mzee Ali (89 years) from Ikwiriri received occasional visits from his daughter, who brought food and water. At some point he stayed alone for five days with hardly anything to eat and drink. According to him, his daughter tried but was struggling to make a living and could not guarantee his care. Eventually, he went to the hospital and was admitted. The daughter paid for his medication and brought over meals while he was hospitalised.

While this is an exceptional case, bordering on neglect, going hungry was a topic brought up by many older people in diverse living arrangements. However, conditions in our research sites were less dramatic than the precariousness faced by many older people in other parts of Tanzania, as in Kagera, for instance (De Klerk, Chapter Six). Like Mzee Ali, the older people in our study commonly explained that their children and/or siblings tried their best but failed to earn a living. Older people who lived by themselves seemed particularly vulnerable. But the giving and withholding of food, drink and care more generally, points to another aspect of the home as a lived space: the exposure of vulnerabilities and dependencies (Tuedio, 2009, 285) and their resulting power relations.

A few *sina nguvu* women in the study also lived alone and received occasional care from outside. In Bumba the husband of a 98-year-old woman lived with his younger second wife, but visited her now and then. Her grandchildren came for longer stays during school holidays. In Ikwiriri an 81-year-old woman lived alone and received help from her two sisters, who stayed in the same village. Better-off women living on their own in Dar es Salaam and Zanzibar had housemaids and/or grandchildren who came to perform domestic care tasks during the day. If they felt worse, they would ask these helpers or other relatives to spend the night with them. In some cases, as the following example shows, tasks were divided among several relatives: a son's ex-wife came three times a week, and a daughter brought a cooked meal every day.

> Bibi Salha (79 years of age) from Zanzibar suffered from heart and respiration problems. She had a housemaid who came in every day, except Sundays; her grandson and his wife stayed with her on that day. She did not leave the house. She could still go to the toilet and bathe, but sometimes needed support. There was always somebody sleeping in her house: the grandson's mother came one day; the sister's daughter the following day. They helped her go to the toilet at night and to the bath in the morning. They sponged her with hot water. If she felt cold, her son bought Vaseline made from coconut, and they applied it to her whole body.

As these examples show, living arrangements do not necessarily reflect care arrangements. The boundaries between homes are fluid and partly intersecting, especially if observed over time. Whenever older women or men experienced a bout of illness or felt particularly weak, close kin made adjustments in nearly all cases. Some helpers visited more often during the daytime, others came to stay for several weeks or months. Some older men and older women received practical help at the same time from inside and outside the home over an extended period of time. With one exception, these cases were recorded in the cities of Dar es Salaam and Zanzibar, where kin – in contrast to our expectations – had particularly close interactions.

The older person is moved to the home of the caregiver

A closer look inside the homes revealed further spatial and temporal dynamics. In all study sites, older men and women had been moved to new homes in order to receive better care. Two men from Rufiji, for instance, who had been brought to Dar es Salaam for an operation a few years ago, still lived with their sons' families. Both felt quite ambivalent about depending on close kin. As Mzee Salem, 85 years old, explained: '*You don't get what you want in time, until you beg, and sometimes these people, if they don't have anything, they will tell you.*' As I mentioned earlier, hunger was a steady companion for many study participants, especially if their families were struggling to make ends meet. At the same time, Mzee Salem considered himself lucky for receiving help from his children and for being respected by them. Mzee Hamadi, 73 years old, expressed similar feelings. On one hand, he was grateful to his son's family, and especially to his granddaughter who cooked for him during the weekdays. On the other hand, he complained that he could not do much but sit and wait until somebody gives him food. He concluded that he 'did not see the joy of old age'; 82-year-old Mzee Mohammed, who lived with his son's family in Zanzibar, made similar remarks: he found it difficult to be forced to live with relatives who had little to share. One of his problems was diet. His doctor said he should not use salt; but since he had to eat what his daughter-in-law prepared for all of them, he had no option. Another problem was that he had to live on painkillers because they could not afford to bring him to the hospital. And even these medicines had to be stretched out as far as possible. He made a single packet last for at least three weeks.

Similar arrangements were found among the older women. In Bumba and Ikwiriri, three Bibis were brought to live in a house with elderly siblings, an arrangement which has become fairly common (see Chapter Three by Van Eeuwijk). Two Bibis from Rufiji and Pemba came to live with their sons' families in Dar es Salaam. Other older women moved within Zanzibar City to find new homes in the families of sons or daughters. Some of these women were happy with their new arrangements, others simply tried to accept what they could not change. Bibi Khalda (80 years old), who was living with her granddaughters in Zanzibar explained her situation as follows:

I can't help myself anymore. Whatever they say, I accept. I am not clever (*sina udhari*) anymore because cleverness is associated with strength (*nguvu*). If you have enough strength in your body, you will manage to live on your own. You may sweep the floor, cook and clean the compound. If you have no strength, you accept whatever people do. And if you consider the facts, I am without strength.

Similar relationships of dependence, which older people did not always find easy to accept, also existed in homes where older people had lived for many years, but they were more pronounced in homes where older people felt like guests. In some of these arrangements, the adult children made decisions, sometimes consulting the older relative, and sometimes against their wishes, as Pype (see Chapter Two of this volume) has also observed in Kinshasa.

Carescapes

Older people from the rural areas often found it difficult to live in the city. Ten of the study participants went to stay with their children in Dar es Salaam for diagnosis and treatment, but returned after a few months because they felt out of place. Others resisted moving, as the example of Bibi Maryamu from Bumba illustrates.

My daughter Zuhura is the one who does everything in the house. She looks after me. She is like a mother to all of us, including the children. She attends the *shamba*. I don't cook, I don't fetch water and I also don't clean the dishes. When I wake up in the morning, I first pray and then go to the backyard to either rest in the sunshine or sweep the compound, if I feel like it. Sometimes I push myself to go to the fields, but only for pleasure, to see the crops grow. Right now, Zuhura is not around. She has gone to see her children who moved to Dar es Salaam. Her sister Aziza came to stay with us. She lives in Dar but always comes during the agricultural season to plough and work the land we gave her. She has grown rice on her farm, and it will be six months before she goes back to Dar es Salaam where her family lives. She is the one looking after me now. My children in town actually ask me to visit them, but I am very straightforward on this: No! To be honest, I do not

like town life. I know the consequences that I might face
by visiting them.

The consequences Bibi Maryamu feared had to do with witchcraft
accusations against older women and the ways people are buried in
town.[5] Like many other older people in the rural and urban study
sites, Bibi Maryamu contrasted safe and resourceful village life with
dangerous and resource-draining city life. Through direct or indirect
experience, most older people were aware that spending one's life in
the city did not guarantee participation in a better life. Older people
faced many obstacles, even those who were better off. Mzee Nassoro
(88 years old), a former businessman from Dar es Salaam, for instance,
knew that he should receive free treatment according to government
policy, but he had given up trying to request free treatment and focused
instead on raising the money for a much-needed prostate operation.
With the help of his children, and especially his daughter, he had
managed to muster £122 for the operation, which cost £162, but
now he was stuck. Most of the urban *sina nguvu* study participants
had a formal medical diagnosis, but this did not necessarily mean that
they had access to appropriate treatment. Having a pension and/or
membership in an insurance scheme increased the chances of adequate
treatment, as a few exceptional cases demonstrate.

In addition to money, most older people in the *sina nguvu* category
lacked what Mzee Nguzo, also from Dar es Salaam, called 'direction'.
He was 77 years old, could not walk because of swollen legs and a heart
problem, and after three years of hospital visits desperately wanted to
know what was wrong with him.

> I have gone to the hospital several times. They gave me
> medication but they didn't say anything. I can't go anymore
> because I don't know anybody there in Muhimbili Hospital.
> There are good doctors, but I have nobody to direct me.
> I can't see them. I have been going there for three years.
> They tell you where you are sick and where to get medicine.
> I can say: this is the third year, please allow me to see the
> professor who is specialised in bones and can tell me why
> I am failing to walk. But I can't see him, I don't have that
> capacity. The children can drive me there in their car but
> I won't see him. I am a very small person, nobody can
> direct me.

Staying at home, often in considerable pain and anger, is less a choice than a restriction imposed on older people. In both urban and rural areas, older people did not merely feel disconnected from the world of formal medical care, they even felt rejected. As Ferguson (2008,10) has shown for urban Zambians, the experience of rejection was often 'not a matter of being *excluded* from a status to which one had never had a claim, but of being expelled in the sense of being cast out-and-down from that status by the formation of a new (or newly impermeable) boundary'. Becoming old and frail was such a new boundary and frequently resulted in less rather than more formal medical care.

Most *sina nguvu* older people in this study depended on their significant others, whether this was a wife, a child or a sibling, not only for practical domestic care, but also for their livelihoods. Those living in the same home carried much of this burden. Other kin provided care from a distance, contributing money, material help like sugar, soap, or medicines, as well as immaterial support like empathy and advice. Kin-based carescapes expanded from the village to the city, to other regions of Tanzania, neighbouring countries and as far as the United States of America or Oman. Whatever distant caregivers sent home was aimed at strengthening the efforts of those who stayed physically close to their parents.

There was also much visiting between and within rural and urban areas. This was shown earlier in the case of Bibi Maryamu's daughters, and it was also true for Mzee Nassoro, whose wife was trying to earn a living by selling tea, and whose daughter temporarily left her own family to stay with her parents. She supported him in trying to raise funds for his prostate operation. Many similar examples were recorded in all study sites. Older people saw opportunities for a better life opening up through expanding and 'changing webs of kinship' (Alber et al, 2010). They mentioned, among other things, improved access to formal medical information and services, general advice concerning modern ways of living and receiving material gifts and financial support.

The older people greatly appreciated visits, not only from their kin but also from neighbours, friends and former work colleagues. Since they themselves could no longer engage in most community activities, they were happy to receive visitors who kept them informed and thus gave them the opportunity to participate from afar. However, while most study participants kept friendly relations with their neighbours, they made it quite clear that the provision of domestic and personal care, as well as general livelihood, had to come from close kin. Several older men and women explicitly stated that it would be a great shame to ask neighbours for support in these matters.

Similarly, only very few of the frail or disabled older men and women in this study received concrete support from non-governmental, community or faith-based organisations, although many had actively participated in such organisations when they were still mobile (for concrete examples of active participation see Chapter Three by Van Eeuwijk). Older people in Ikwiriri and Bumba who were reached by the eye programme of the Comprehensive Community-Based Rehabilitation Tanzania based in Dar es Salaam, were a rare exception. All older people considered religious faith and prayers as a source of strength and comfort, even if they could not walk to the church or mosque and take part in collective prayers and ceremonies. But while lived religion was clearly a shaping force in old-age care as well as for the younger generations, concrete help from such organisations rarely materialised in older people's everyday experiences.

Conclusions

Based on the evidence presented in this chapter, I have argued that an embodiment perspective helps us to get closer to older people's everyday experiences of care in rural and urban Tanzania, but also yields more general information (see Becker, 1994). Such a perspective shows that the lived body gains in importance as older people lose the strength to take care of themselves and perform domestic and livelihood activities. Older people become often painfully aware of their bodies' spatial and temporal dimensions, and may experience them as adversaries, or even agents that take control over their selves. Vulnerability of body and self becomes older people's ever present companion. This does not mean that they become victims, rather the physical changes in their bodies surely affect their 'internal agency' (ways of experiencing the world) and their 'external agency' (actual interactions with people, places and events) (see Emirbayer and Mische, 1998, 973). In other words, they are forced to reorder their relationships to their bodies and selves, as well as to other people, places and events.

In this process, the home as a lived space becomes a key site of old-age care. Its material form varied greatly within and across the rural and urban research areas covered in this study. A systematic inquiry into what constitutes, in a material sense, a 'good' versus 'bad' home for frail and disabled older people, would certainly yield valuable insights, given, also, the increased global interest in the topic of 'ageing in place' (Vasunilashorn et al, 2012). In the United States and in Europe, politicians, activists and gerontologists now consider 'ageing in place' as a goal or even a new paradigm. They promote the design of policies and programmes that would enable older people to continue living independent lives in their homes, supported by services and technologies to compensate for loss of strength and mobility.

The emphasis in this chapter has been on the home in the sense of belonging to a 'field of interrelatedness' and 'intimate involvements' (Tuedio, 2009). When their physical strength, and thus their mobility, decreases, older people's engagement with other people becomes increasingly restricted to close kin, such as spouses, siblings, adult children and grandchildren. As the discussion of the three most prevalent care arrangements has shown, the boundaries among homes were fluid and partly intersecting, especially if observed over time. Especially in Dar es Salaam and Zanzibar, close relatives living in different homes contributed to the care of older men or women. This was less the case in the scattered rural settlements. As older, but especially younger, people moved within and across rural and urban sites, this field of interrelatedness was continuously reconfigured.

In this process, connections with formal medical carescapes opened and closed. The younger generation encouraged their parents to seek professional help in the city. With their financial, logistical and practical support, several older people succeeded in having their eyes, *busha*, or prostate operated on in specialised health facilities. Others got stuck due to financial problems or because they lacked 'directions', even when they had lived in the city their entire lives. Still others returned home after receiving the diagnosis that they suffered from an incurable disease like Parkinson's. In all research sites, older people reported experiences of rejection by formal medical care providers. Such negative interactions can be at least partly explained by the fact that health care services in Tanzania are primarily geared towards young children and pregnant mothers. When a person reaches the age of 60+, she may face a new boundary when she approaches formal medical services, even though the Tanzanian government has issued an exemption policy for older people (URT, 2003).

A remarkable finding of this study is that only close kin – in a social rather than geographical sense – are involved in the provision of personal care and livelihood. Neighbours, friends and tenants sometimes assist with advice, comfort, or practical help. Asking them for more intimate involvement would be considered shameful, not only for the older person but also for his or her close kin. An exception to this rule seems to be the employment of paid helpers (*dada*). Although the boundary between a paid helper and a foster child was not always clear in this study, this development deserves further inquiry as it may present a culturally accepted way of alleviating the care burden of close kin (see also Van der Geest, Chapter One and Van Eeuwijk, Chapter Three).

In summary, this study shows that the everyday care experiences of frail or disabled elderly people in Tanzania are anchored in the home, where diverse carescapes intersect. The boundaries among these care spaces are shifting, but thus far close kin have played the most active roles in shaping these boundaries, while the government and non-governmental and faith-based organisations, as well as private actors hardly engage in the care of frail or disabled old people. To my surprise, these general principles applied in all four study sites, although the details of how they played out differed.

Notes

[1] The Swahili term *busha* refers both to a groin hernia or a hydrocele. In areas like the Rufiji District, where *Lymphatic filiarisis* is highly endemic, the hydrocele is most likely a clinical manifestation of this disease which is transmitted by mosquitoes (Ntuli et al, 2009).

[2] 'Mzee' and 'Bibi' are respectful Swahili terms of address for an older man and woman, respectively.

[3] This chapter refers to but does not elaborate on the temporal dimension, which is of course inherent in the ageing experience and deserves a full inquiry of its own.

[4] See Acknowledgements; this chapter draws on the PhD projects of Vendelin T. Simon (2012) on Rufiji, Jana Gerold (2012) on Dar es Salaam, Andrea Grolimund on Dar es Salaam/USA and Sandra Staudacher on Zanzibar/Oman.

[5] In certain parts of Tanzania and in other areas of Africa, older women are often accused of witchcraft (see Mesaki, 2009 and Pype, Chapter Two in this volume). With regard to burials in town, many people were concerned that their graves would be disturbed, for instance by construction work.

Acknowledgements

I gratefully acknowledge the contributions of all research team members and thank all the institutions, the local authorities, the research assistants, and especially the study participants for their support. The research team for the first project 'From "Cure to Care" among the Elderly: Old Age Vulnerability in Tanzania' (2008–11) consisted of members of the Institute of Social Anthropology, University of Basel, Switzerland (Dr Peter van Eeuwijk, leader; Prof Dr Brigit Obrist,

advisor; Jana Gerold, PhD student), the Department of Sociology/
Anthropology, University of Dar es Salaam, Tanzania (Dr Joyce Nyoni,
country coordinator; Vendelin T. Simon, PhD student) and the Ifakara
Health Institute, Tanzania (Dr Flory Kessy, Dr Honorati Masanja,
Siegbert Mrema). The research team for the second project 'Ageing,
Agency and Health in Urbanizing Tanzania' (2012–16) involved
members of the Institute of Social Anthropology, University of Basel,
Switzerland (Prof Dr Brigit Obrist, leader; Dr Peter van Eeuwijk, senior
researcher; Andrea Grolimund, PhD student; and Sandra Staudacher,
PhD student) and the Department of Sociology/Anthropology,
University of Dar es Salaam, Tanzania (Dr Joyce Nyoni, Tanzanian
principal investigator; Dr Vendelin T. Simon, senior researcher). The
interviews were carried out by the PhD students and their research
assistants. Both projects were funded by the Swiss National Science
Foundation, received ethical clearance from the NIMR, Tanzania and
a research permit from COSTECH, Tanzania.

References
Alber, E, Häberlein, T, Jeannett, M, 2010, Changing webs of kinship:
Spotlights on West Africa, *Africa Spectrum* 45, 3, 43–67
Appadurai, A, 2005, *Modernity at large: Cultural dimensions of globalization.*
Minneapolis, MN: University of Minnesota Press
Becker, G, 1994, The oldest old: Autonomy in the face of frailty,
Journal of Aging Studies 8, 1, 59–76
Cresswell, T, 2004, *Place: A short introduction,* Hoboken: Wiley-
Blackwell
Emirbayer, M, Mische, A, 1998, What is agency?, *American Journal of
Sociology* 103, 4, 962–1023
Ferguson, JG, 2008, Global disconnect: Abjection and the aftermath of
modernism, in P Geschiere, B Meyer, P Pels (eds) *Readings in modernity
in Africa*, pp 8–16, London: The International Africa Institute
Gerold, J, 2012, Full of life: Old age and care in urban Dar es Salaam,
Unpublished PhD Dissertation, Basel: University of Basel
Hitchcock, M, 2002, Zanzibar Stone Town joins the imagined
community of World Heritage Sites, *International Journal of Heritage
Studies* 8, 2, 153–66
Jackson, JE, 1994, 'After a while no one believes you': Real and unreal
pain, in M-J Del Vecchio Good, PE Brodwin, BJ Good, A Kleinman
(eds) *Pain as human experience: An anthropological perspective*, pp 138–68,
Berkeley, CA: University of California Press

Johansson, H, Saarikangas, K, 2009, Introduction: Ambivalent homes, in H Johansson, K Saarikangas (eds) *Homes in transformation: Dwelling, moving, belonging*, pp 9–35, Helsinki: Finnish Literature Society

Merleau-Ponty, M, 1962, *The phenomenology of perception*, New York: Humanities Press [Original: *Phénoménologie de la Perception*, Paris: Gallimard, 1945]

Mesaki, S, 2009, The tragedy of ageing: Witch killings and poor governance among the Sukuma, in L Haram, CB Yamba (eds) *Dealing with uncertainty in contemporary African lives*, pp 72–90, Uppsala: Nordiska Afrikainstitutet

NBS (National Bureau of Statistics), 2013, *Tanzania in figures 2012*, Dar es Salaam: Ministry of Finance

Ntuli, MW, Lazarus, W, Mwingira, U, Mwakitalu, E, Makene, C, Kabali, C, Mackenzie, C, 2009, Eliminating LF: A progress report from Tanzania, *Journal of Lymphoedema* 4, 2–4

Obrist, B, 2006, *Struggling for health in the city: An anthropological inquiry of health, vulnerability and resilience in Dar es Salaam, Tanzania*, Bern: Peter Lang

Seamon, D, 2014, Physical and virtual environments: Meanings of place and space, in BA Boyt Schell, G Gillen, ME Scaffa (eds) *Willard and Spackman's occupational therapy*, 12th edn, pp 202–14, Baltimore: Lipincott, Williams and Wilkins

Simon, VT, 2012, Ageing, health and care in rural Tanzania, Unpublished PhD Dissertation, Basel: University of Basel

Toombs, K, 1993, *The meaning of illness: A phenomenological account of the different perspectives of physician and patient,* Dordrecht: Kluwer

Toombs, K, 2001, Introduction: Phenomenology and medicine, in K Toombs (ed) *Handbook of phenomenology and medicine*, pp 1–26, Dordrecht: Kluwer

Tuedio, J, 2009, Ambiguities in the locus of home: Exilic life and the space of belonging, in H Johansson, K Saarikangas (eds) *Homes in transformation: Dwelling, moving, belonging*, pp 284–310, Helsinki: Finnish Literature Society

UN-HABITAT, 2010, *Citywide action plan for upgrading unplanned and unserviced settlements in Dar es Salaam*, Nairobi: UN-HABITAT

URT (United Republic of Tanzania), Ministry of Labour, Youth Development and Sports, 2003, *National ageing policy*, Dar es Salaam, Tanzania: Ministry of Labour, Youth Development and Sports

Vasunilashorn, S, Steinman, B, Liebig, PS, Pynoos, J, 2012, Ageing in place: Evolution of a research topic whose time has come, *Journal of Ageing Research,* Article ID 120952, doi:10.1155/2012/120952

FIVE

Care and identity in rural Malawi

Emily Freeman

Introduction

Political and academic concern that care for older adults in Sub-Saharan Africa is insufficient and under strain in light of changing demography and society is long standing (UN, 1982), but poorly set out. Questions remain unanswered: What is meant by 'care' and what is the care that older adults need? Do (all) older adults want this (undefined) care? If they do, when do they want it and from whom? Much of the established discourse implies incapacity in older age, a burden of care to be shouldered by family, and homogenised 'elderly people' who want, and sometimes successfully motivate, care.

In 2008 I started a conversation with older men and women in rural Malawi about their experiences of ageing. Caregiving and -receipt was a recurring narrative in our discussions, and at the heart of their understandings of older age. 'Care', 'help', 'assistance', 'support', 'looking after' and 'keeping', were used interchangeably in conversations to refer to a wide variety of practices, from assistance with washing, mobility and feeding ('basic activities of daily living') and farm- and housework ('instrumental activities of daily living'), to gifts of maize, clothes and money, as well as vigilance to need, for example, by regularly visiting to monitor a person's welfare as they aged. Some older adults were receiving this broadly defined care, and from those from whom they expected it; some were not, left without care because of poverty, HIV, poor planning or just bad luck:

> A lot of people passed away, so the ones who are left behind cannot care for the old people: that old person complains, 'It would be better God took me.' Then there are other old people who have children, who have gone to school and are working, so when that old man is ageing, the children assist him. And there are other old people who suffer, even though they have children. (Estina, female, 55)

As might be expected, and found in other settings (see Van der Geest, Chapter One), care was inconsistently presented, even within a single interview. Sometimes participants would talk about the care they received and at other times deny receiving any help at all. Sometimes participants centred discussions of care only on the giving and receiving of larger resources (for example maize, school fees, building or repairing a house, digging a latrine) or on farming assistance given by someone who would not eventually share the produce. At other times smaller resources (salt, analgesics, a few Kwacha) or help with housework (fetching water, cooking, sweeping) were included in conversations about care. Sometimes participants did not mention non-financial care if it was given by or to their parent or child, but at other times, it was these relationships that made the care salient and the subject of conversation. Assistance for the sick or frail, such as help with bathing or with getting around was usually always referred to as care, but if the assistance was given by a spouse, or was received by a participant in response to older age rather than (non-age related) illness, it was not readily discussed unless we asked about that specific care practice. How and if care was discussed by participants differed depending on the context of the care in question (whether it was care given or received by the participant, the type of care, the actors involved, the circumstances in which it was given) but also on the context of the conversation: that is, what else we had discussed that day.

Despite these differences in receipt of care and the way that care was (not) discussed, there were patterns in the way participants used the concept of care in their conversations. This chapter focuses on those patterns. It argues that research conversations about care became a discursive space in which participants explored what the giving, receiving and needing of care meant for their sense of selves as they aged. All participants presented their experiences of care in ways which they understood would demonstrate positive self-identities. They talked much less about availability of care, and much more about what the giving and receiving of care 'said' about them.

Drawing on sociological theories of identity, this chapter considers the implications of the meanings associated with different types of care for older adults' age-related identity scripts. Receipt of care in response to vulnerability or from those who could not easily provide it was framed with reference to overwhelmingly negative, body-centred understandings of old age that presented a challenge to older men and women's central identities as 'adults' – defined by participants as valid members of the social world. Emphasis on self-care and reciprocity in older adults' narratives can thus be considered strategies to maintain positive 'adult' identities.

The implication of care for participants' identities was a salient part of their wider ageing experiences, but is infrequently discussed in the political and academic conversation around ageing and care in Africa. Anthropological work excepted (for example Cattell, 2002; Van der Geest, 2002a; 2002b), much of the research on African ageing carried out in the social sciences since the late 1980s, primarily concerned with producing insights to inform policy responses to 'the problem of ageing' in the face of under-explored social change, has focused on *provision* of care for older adults: whether or not older adults are (still) receiving care (Stroeken, 2002). Evidence and explanatory frameworks that take into account motivations for providing and receiving care and older adults' strategies to respond and adapt to their changing situations are needed (Aboderin, 2004; Ferreira, 1999; Peil, 1987). This chapter contributes to attempts to incorporate older adults' *experiences* of care – needed, given and received – more fully within representations of ageing in Africa.

Methodology

I spent 12 months between 2008 and 2010 living with and talking to older adults in Malawi in order to understand their experiences of growing old and of HIV infection. Constructivist grounded theory (Charmaz, 2006) was used to carry out the study, privileging what older adults themselves presented as the salient elements of their experiences. Our conversations included relationships, politics, death, sex, love, having HIV and growing old. This chapter presents my analytical account of their understandings and experiences of care in older age.

In-depth interviews were the primary method of generating data to access people's thoughts on unobservable, multi-layered, complex and emotionally-charged experiences and behaviours (Sommer and Sommer, 1991). Participants were initially recruited from those who had taken part in the Malawi Longitudinal Study of Families and Health (Anglewicz et al, 2009). Knowing something about potential participants before approaching them meant that an ongoing theoretical sampling strategy could be used, with each person recruited based on characteristics (for example, age, HIV, gender, living arrangements) likely to be important for exploring analytical ideas being developed about data generated. Further participants were recruited from the families of existing participants' (parents, children and spouses), HIV support groups and the local area (for example, healers).

This chapter draws on data from interviews (n=135) with 44 men and women living in approximately 25 small, rural villages in or close to Balaka District, southern Malawi. They were relatively evenly spread between approximate ages 50 and 90 years. It is a weakness of the study, aiming as it does to prioritise participants' concerns and perspectives rather than mine, that this chronological age range had little significance for them: many did not know their birth year and some did not self-define as 'older'. Nevertheless, this sampling frame meant that a wide variety of experiences and understandings of ageing could be elicited from a population that represents that which policy makers and much of the academy refer to when they talk about old age in Africa (WHO, 2001). Although approximations of chronological age are given alongside quotations reproduced in this chapter, participants' understandings of their age were used in the analysis.

Interviews presented here were carried out in Chiyao or Chichewa with the help of local research assistants between March 2009 and May 2010. Most participants were visited three or four times for audio-recorded interviews typically lasting one or two hours, although some were much longer. Analysis of these interviews was additionally informed by analysis of data from observations made during visits to participants' homes throughout fieldwork, group interviews with older adults with HIV in Balaka (n=3) and initial exploratory in-depth interviews with older adults (n=42) conducted between June and August 2008 in all three regions of Malawi.

The corporality of care in Balaka

Balaka is one of the poorest regions of Malawi, one of the poorest countries in the world (UNDP, 2010). Almost 85 per cent of Malawians, and over 90 per cent of Malawians aged 50 and older, live in rural areas (NSO, 2008) as smallholder subsistence farmers (Chintsanya et al, 2010). Livelihoods in Balaka centre on self-sufficiency in maize production. They featured heavily in older adult's narratives about a wide range of issues, including care.

The dominance of livelihoods in research conversations reflects daily routines, but also high levels of food insecurity and widespread poverty. Along with their families, all participants experienced food shortages, at least during the annual 'hunger season'. Almost all older men and women continued to farm, some supplementing this with inconsistent and modest earnings from the sale of cash crops of cotton and tobacco, reed mats they had woven or snacks they had made (older women only). Two older men variably ran businesses in the trading centre while their families farmed – a tea shop and an 'electronics shop' with a refrigerator selling cold drinks – although these were a no more reliable source of income.

There is little formal care provision in Malawi. Typically, when individuals lack the capacity for (mainly) agricultural self-sufficiency, temporarily or permanently, the family is called upon to provide care. As explored in this volume by De Klerk (Chapter Six) and Van der Geest (Chapter One) in Tanzania and Ghana, participants' caregiving relationships were not innate, based on pre-determined roles, but continually evolving social processes formed and shaped through daily interactions. Their experiences and expectations of receiving care were situated within a complex web of support networks, based on a principle, if not practice, of reciprocity.

Care was discussed in the context of this socio-economic structure of subsistence agriculture and familial safety nets. In older adults' narratives, care implies survival through providing for oneself (self-care) and for those less able to support themselves. It is exclusively discussed in terms of the provision, need and receipt of physical assistance rather than emotional support. The body is central to such care. In the absence of other opportunities for employment in this rural setting, for both younger and older adults the body's capacity for physical labour – farm work, housework, or 'bedwork' (marital sex) – is essential to be able to care for oneself and secure reciprocal care from others: 'For your daily life, you have to work. You have to work for the life you are living. There is a saying which goes "He who does not work should not eat"'(Lyness, male, 68).

The body's capacity for all types of work is determined by its fluids. All fluids (blood, sweat, ejaculate) contain a life force – a quality of 'being alive', translated as 'power' or 'strength'. This life force is strongest in the blood. Subsequently, participants typically referred to all bodily fluids and the body's power as 'blood'.

The life course is understood to be a linear trajectory of diminishing blood (power/strength) until death. However physical labour requires a lot of strength so 'uses up' an individual's broadly finite store of blood, hastening their decline. Support relationships involve the giving and receiving of blood. Bodies without sufficient blood cannot perform self-care, nor can they care for others. However, since care is reciprocal, as long as some of a body's blood has been used caring for others, in principle that individual can expect to receive care.

Although older adults called upon extended family, friends or community groups at times of crisis (for example bereavement, severe but short illness, theft of maize), adult children[1] and spouses were the most important exchange relations when longer-term, regular care in older age was needed. Van der Geest observes in Ghana 'there may be some rules about who should care for the old, but that does not yet predict unambiguously who will actually do the caring' (Van der Geest, 2002a, 23). Similarly, while these relations did not necessarily provide care to participants, it was these relations – or the absence of them – that they referred to most often when discussing the management of current or expected age-related declines in ability to work. They prioritised these relations in research conversations because of the level of investment they had made in them – or could have made in them. This principle of care 'investments' – food provided, physical care given, money spent – played out daily and over years, has been described in many African settings (for example Cattell, 1990; Schatz and Ogunmefun, 2007; Hoffman, Chapter Seven; De Klerk, Chapter Six; and Van der Geest, Chapter One). Here, investments were explicitly body-centred, tied to exchanges of blood.

In participants' narratives conception, pregnancy and childbirth are presented as having used a substantial amount of a woman's finite blood (and in the giving of semen, a smaller quantity of a man's blood). Children are expected to 'repay' the strength contained within this blood by caring for their mothers in later life:

> When I am careful with [maize] it takes me through the year. But if things are not well, it does not last me a year...I tell my children that my food is finished...and the children assist me...Because I know that they are the ones I shared my blood with. I tell them because there are no other people who can assist me apart from them. They understand because I am their mother, I gave birth to them and I suffered a lot for them. (Lizzie, female, late 50s)

In participants' narratives, however, those who have not made sufficient investments cannot expect to receive support from their children in older age. Robertson's case highlights this well. Recently re-married, Robertson was living in his wife's village, a few miles from his first marital home. He saw little of his children, who had yet to visit him at his new home. He explained that although he might like to, he knew he could not complain about this and did not expect them to care for him in the future because, having left their mother and them while they were young, he had not met the conditions of reciprocity:

No, the children I have…don't come to visit me here…
No, when I go there to visit them they are happy, when I
ask them why they are not visiting me here they say they
will come, 'sometime'. I stop it there. I did my job, that's
all. I produced them [but didn't raise them]…It would be
different if I had paid *lobola*[2] – I would be worried then
because they would be living with me here [and receiving
support] and if they would not support me *then*, I would
be worried. (Robertson, male, 80s)

Robertson wasn't concerned. He had his new wife, a strong and vibrant
village head, should he need care in the future. Indeed, marriage is
important for giving and receipt of non-intimate and intimate care.
In contrast to caring in Tanzania discussed in this volume, this elder-
to-elder care was a well-established social norm, presented as the
preferred option when older age care was needed by older men and
women as well as their children (see Van Eeuwijk, Chapter Three).
While unmarried or recently-married participants discussed the benefit
of new partnerships for securing care in older age, it was longstanding
spouses who were most prized, specifically because of the length of time
over which bodily investments in the relationship – years of farming,
cooking, sharing sexual fluids (see Freeman and Coast, 2014) – could be
made. For example, Rhoda explained that her older husband's declining
productivity was a result of having shared his blood with her and her
co-wife and was quick to affirm her intention to reciprocate his care:

[My husband] is not working much as compared to those
days when he was energetic…The time he was coming [to
marry me] I had no kitchen but he constructed the kitchen,
toilet and put up the fence. But nowadays he cannot
manage to do that. He is unable to provide us with money.
I understand the situation is that he is ageing…so I just
say let us just be keeping each other. (Rhoda, female, 56)

Both older men and women provided personal care for their spouses
when it was needed. Some of this care, such as bathing, involved intimate
contact with naked bodies. Participants' sexualised understandings of
their bodies partly underpinned their universal preference for spousal
rather than child carers, and then gender-matched carers, regardless
of investment made in relationships.

The corporality of identity

The familial support system was, however, rarely enacted as smoothly, deterministically or reciprocally as this. Children and spouses died, leaving older adults without the support which they expected to receive, as well as heartbroken. Relations contested investments made and support due. Children migrated and 'forgot' their parents. Families argued and broke apart. Participants bemoaned adult children who through habit or laziness still relied on them for support. Given high levels of food scarcity and poverty, care was only given or expected from kin who could afford the resources or time to provide it, regardless of investments made. Moreover when those who were providing care discussed their motivation, love and familial bond was as important as any sense of investment or payback. But while the rhetoric of blood given and repaid did not always line up with the practicalities of everyday life, it is this body-centred understanding of care that underpinned its consequences for older adults' identities.

For participants, the body's ability to perform care – that is, to support oneself and others through the various practices outlined above (farm work, housework, personal care and so on) – demonstrated an individual's status as an 'adult': a socially-valid person. As observed in other settings (Comaroff and Comaroff, 2001; Guillette, 1992; Cattell, 2002), in the social and structural context of rural Balaka, an individual not only secures their and their dependants' survival through performing care, they produce their entitlement to membership of the social world of 'adults'. Those who are not able to perform care are excluded. These individuals, rarely young, were defined in opposition, as 'children'. The production of the adult identity is therefore embodied in the act of care.

Here sociological theories of identity provide a useful analytical lens.[3] Role identity theory, the theory of 'possible selves' (Markus and Nurius, 1986) and 'identity control' theory (Burke, 2006) encourage us to consider *how* performing care and adulthood are linked for older adults and *why* identities are so important in shaping experiences of care. They inspire reflection on the ways participants maintained positive identities even as they described age-related changes that would challenge those identities, extending existing academic understandings of ageing and care.

According to role identity theory, people derive individual-level social identities from the roles they play within the social structure (for example, teacher, mother), based on the socially-constructed shared meanings and expectations associated with those roles and their performance (such as 'knowledgeable' for the teacher identity, 'caring' for the mother identity) (Burke and Tully, 1977). These role expectations form a set of 'identity standards' that guide behaviour. That is, 'in order to be (some identity), one must act like (some identity)' (Burke and Reitzes, 1981, 90). This process is reciprocal. Individuals classify themselves as having a particular identity based on their behaviours, and behave in ways which they believe reinforce and confirm that identity.

A role identity is arrived at when:

- an individual identifies with a socially-recognised role;
- others identify them as occupying that role;
- they achieve gratification by performing in that role; and
- the demands of a particular situation make enacting the role socially appropriate and appreciated (McCall and Simmons, 1966).

Having a particular identity involves coordinating and negotiating with individuals with related, complementary or counter-roles (for example, teacher–pupil, mother–child). It is only during this interaction that an individual identifies with their role identity (Burke and Reitzes, 1981; Stets and Burke, 2000).

In participants' narratives, to have the role identity 'adult', one must act in ways that are interpreted by oneself and observers as being able to care for oneself (at least partially, in not being wholly dependent), and as being able to care for others (at least partially, in making some contribution towards others' wellbeing). Since physical labour – 'work' – is understood to be the only behaviour available through which to perform care, for participants, to be an adult an individual's behaviour must be recognisably work: working is the identity standard for the role identity of an adult. The performance of care through physical work therefore reflected and shaped participants' identities as 'adults'.

Participants drew on their interactions with others in the context of performing care to establish their adult role identities. In the following excerpt, Lyness refers to the reactions of those around him to confirm that his behaviour demonstrates his identity as an independent, contributing – caring – adult. He distances himself from the counter-role occupied by those 'who don't work':

> I am old and people respect me. Other people take me as
> an adult, not an old man, because I am working and have
> power...You know I am working...This makes me have
> some money to support myself and my family. There are

others who don't work but are staying at home...They may look older than me [because] they don't have proper care... Because I am working, my friends look at me as someone different. When they come to me, they know that they can ask for help. (Lyness, male, 68)

Individuals have numerous positive identities, and rely on them at different times as a particular identity becomes relevant in a social situation (becomes 'activated') (Burke, 2006). Older men and women in Balaka presented themselves as occupying a range of identities: fathers, daughters, good Muslims, competent lovers, jokers. However, the 'adult' identity and the behaviours understood as standard for that identity (bodily capacity and production) dominated research conversations about ageing. Of all participants' identities, the 'adult' identity formed a central, salient identity in our conversations, activated by talking about needing and receiving care.

Threat to the adult identity presented by needing and receiving care in old age

Through decreasing blood, ageing was understood to undermine an individual's ability to care for themselves or others. At its culmination, this inability produced dependent behaviour that, for participants, was incompatible with the adult identity. The 'childlike' old become 'useless':

The aged walk like children, senseless things. Yes, they don't take care of themselves and we take care of them. To say let us take care of the aged, because she is now useless. So we fetch some water for her to bathe. Cook the food and give to her so she doesn't get worried...[At that stage] there are a lot of problems you face: you crawl and at times you are pushed by children, because you are useless. (Ethel, female, late 80s/early 90s)

Throughout this volume the gradual decline in bodily strength (De Klerk, Chapter Six) and ability to work (Obrist, Chapter Four) are presented as key experiences of ageing. The following interview extract and field note highlight the process of non-adult identity formation associated with these experiences. Wyson's mental and physical health had declined. Aged around 85 he lived with his sister, her husband and children. He presents his behaviour in ways that mirror their observations, highlighting how his inability to care for himself through farm- or housework removes him from the social world of adults ('men').

> On this first visit to his home we were greeted by his sister. We explained we had come to visit Wyson to talk with him about our research. She seemed amused that we thought we would learn from him and warned us that he was 'just like a child'. Other members of the household came over to talk to us. His 48-year-old nephew was concerned for our research, telling us we would learn more by speaking to another member of the household. I am sure that Wyson, sitting close-by, could hear this conversation.

> *I:* So, at first you should please tell more about yourself.
> *P:* My family ended some time back. And at this time I have nothing to do with marriage. Currently it is my sister and my in-law who are taking care of me.
> *I:* So what do you do here at home?
> *P:* …I do nothing. I stopped my hands. I can't do any task.
> *I:* OK. So in this community, do they use you as a very old person to perform some duties?
> *P:* I do nothing.
> [Participant's sister (S), calling across the compound: He does nothing!]
> *P:* I just stay.
> *I:* Mmm
> *S:* I am just feeding him!
> *I* [To S]: Would you please allow that all the questions should be answered by your brother?
> *S:* OK
> *I:* Do you farm?
> *P:* No, I don't cultivate, I stopped.
> *I:* Do you do any business?
> *P:* Nothing. Aah, I just stay idle.
> *I:* May be cooking when your sister is not here?
> *P:* No, I can't.
> *I:* OK. Do you take yourself as an old person?
> *P:* I am an old person, no doubt about that.
> *I:* OK. Thank you, Grandfather. So since that time you were born, up to this time, what has changed on this earth, in the world, but also in your life?

> *P:*...What has changed is that I am not able to do things.
> I am not a man enough.

On hearing his family's description of him prior to the interview, Wyson immediately directs the conversation to his inability to work, evaluating his behaviour as falling short of the identity standard for an adult – 'a man'. He returned to his physical ability and inability regularly in subsequent conversations, reflecting the salience of these corporeal changes and their meanings to his identity.

For participants autonomy and ownership were the domains of the adult. Participants understood inability to care for oneself in old age to undermine these basic privileges. They frequently commented on the powerlessness of the very old who 'just stay', awaiting care. Wyson's loss of agency characterised his experience of receiving care from his sister: 'There is a difference. This time there are rules. Those days I was the one making rules, [but now] I cannot, it is not my house. There is no way you can order them to give you water to bathe.'

Other participants simply feared this experience:

> [Getting older] is not good because you become a child, when a person is old they just wait to be fed, people to do things for them. Eeh, it is a bad thing, because you become a child, and the things you used to do when you were young, you cannot do them because you do not have the strength...it will be painful...because a person can do something for you which you didn't want, in so doing you start remembering what you used to do in the past while you were strong. (Ethel, female, late 80s/early 90s)

Ability to perform care and avoid childlike dependence is universally referenced in participants' descriptions of a good or a bad old age.

> A good old age, I do put it at the stage, where one is still able to do some work, not just being kept in the house, that kind of old age is not good...We had a certain old man, he just died recently. He couldn't walk out of the house by himself, he couldn't do things on his own. His grandchildren would pick him [up] to go outside to have the sun, he could be crying. So when we saw that the old man, [we thought] that old age is too much. He was not eating by himself because he was just like a child. He was

just like a child, he could even fear a goat, when it is [only] a goat! (Alick, male, early 50s)

More intensive physical care needed by older adults who cannot care for themselves tests the strength of reciprocal support. Participants expected that carers in this situation would be more likely to demonstrate feeling burdened by providing inadequate care:

> *I:* Have you ever seen somebody very old who was being taken care of?
> *P:* Yes, my grandmother.
> *I:* How old was she?
> *P:* I don't know...but she reached a point that when she has slept she could not wake up alone.
> *I:* How was she taken care of?
> *P:* She could be carried from the house to the veranda, cooking for her.
> *I:* Bathing her?
> *P:* Yes, and washing her clothes.
> *I:* The time these people were helping your grandmother, were they happy or not?
> *P:* They could complain because they were troubled.
> *I:* What were they saying?
> *P:*...Sometimes you can tell because of how the people are behaving. Let's say the time she wants something, you found that there was no one to provide that thing. (Susan, female, mid-60s)

Exceeded investments for intimate and non-intimate care are most likely when the only carer available is from outside the immediate family. Although a number of participants spoke with tenderness about having given care to friends (for example, one participant talked of caring for her best friend before she died of AIDS, another of how, as a younger man, he had provided intimate care for his former employer, whom he continued to respect) they rarely ground narratives about receiving care in their own experiences as caregivers. As Obrist observes (Chapter Four), participants instead reported that prolonged dependency on those outside the family would become socially unacceptable:

> There is an age where a person can be respected, even though they are old. Mainly that will happen when they

have children who can support them. Even if they become very old, they will have the support they need. But if you don't have children to support you, and you depend on other people to help you, you don't get respected. (Fiskani, male, 61)

Nevertheless, while exceeded reciprocity was more likely with non-familial carers, for some participants, reliance on children presented an equally grave threat to adulthood. In South Africa Hoffman describes how older adults provide care for their children regardless of context (Chapter Seven). Similarly in Balaka, older adults reported that younger generations should always take precedence over their parents. For them, a good parent – and a provident adult – first cares for their children, enabling them to 'develop', and when they can no longer do so, takes less blood from their children than they have given to them. Demanding intensive care from children was understood to prevent them from working to improve their own lives and was incompatible with the behaviour held within the adult identity standard.

Of all the behaviours compromised by the ageing body, it is incontinence and inability to provide intimate personal care for oneself that presented the greatest threat to the adult identity. That receipt of intimate care can undermine an individual's respect (Van der Geest, 2002b) and status as a complete social being (Luborsky, 1994; Schröder-Butterfill and Fithry, 2014) has been observed in a wide range of settings. In the UK, Julia Twigg has observed how personal care 'marks the boundary of the wholly personal and individual in modern life. Having to receive help in such areas transgresses social boundaries and undermines one's status as an adult. These things are normally only done for babies' (Twigg, 2006, 122).

In participants' narratives the meanings assigned to the receipt of intimate care are not compatible with the identity standard of the adult. Need for such care is evidence of lacking the lowest level of self-sufficiency. It requires a level of support transfers that go beyond those covered by the covenant of reciprocity: at this stage, blood received will certainly be greater than the blood given throughout the life course.

The childlike 'possible self'

While some participants were in good health and produced food and resources that supported themselves and dependants, others struggled with limited eyesight, poor mobility and *nyamakazi* (rheumatism, neuralgia or sciatica, understood to be caused by blood drying), and were more frequently the recipients than providers of care. However, these participants presented their experiences inconsistently. The following extracts are from a single conversation with Rhoda. Here, as across a further three interviews, her narrative oscillates between losing physical strength and continued ability to work:

> *P:* Sometimes I have malaria, plus *nyamakazi* which prevents me from weaving mats. But it affects me more early in the morning.
> *I:* What have you been doing during this week?
> *P:* I was doing some housework, like sweeping on the ground, cooking relish, nsima, taking water from the borehole.
>
> …
>
> *I:* What has changed in your life over the last 20 years?
> *P:* My body. The changes which I have seen are that I am failing to do hard work, and when I force myself to do it I become sick…I am failing to do the work…It pains me much.
>
> …
>
> *I:* How do you feel about getting older?
> *P:* I feel good about getting older with my husband, because we work together in our works…I am looking forward to it because I take care of myself and my husband.
>
> …
>
> *P:* Paining headache, I fail to work most of the times because of that problem.
>
> …
>
> *I:* So what do you think is the best time of life for a person?
> *P:* It's when you are a girl or when you have two children. Because you have full blood in your body. (Rhoda, female, 56)

Rhoda's narrative is common. At some point during conversations all participants reported working. This was essential for securing their survival, even when care was available. However, their narratives can also be understood to reflect their active negotiation of the challenges to their adult identities which they experienced or expected from their ageing bodies.

Despite universal understanding of the inevitability of bodily decline and dependency in old age among participants, no participants identified with the 'child' identity counter-role; even Wyson was not consistent in reports that he was 'finished'. Instead, it presented for all participants a 'possible self' (Markus and Nurius, 1986): an identity they may have in the future when the meanings of their behaviour cannot be aligned with those held in the 'adult' identity standard.

Although only a few participants had seen childlike old people first hand, all feared this future for themselves. Fear of this possible self was fear of losing oneself; passing beyond what it meant to be 'them': 'In the future *I will not be the same person*. I will *not be able to do the things* I am doing now. Time will elapse. By that I mean I will be a very old man' (Rabson, male, 75 (emphasis added)).

This period of incapacity in old age has been usefully conceptualised for western ageing experiences as a 'black hole', exerting a gravitational pull on those too close to this life phase (Gilleard and Higgs, 2010, 125). The metaphor certainly accords with participants' interview narratives in which they appeared to consistently 'pull back' from reporting need for care.

According to the theory of possible selves, individuals are motivated to avoid negative future identities and pursue positive future identities. Possible selves thereby become incentives that guide behaviours, thoughts and strategies (Markus and Nurius, 1986). Older adults in this study were motivated to maintain their adult identities and avoid the 'black hole' of the childlike possible self.

They employed two discursive strategies to do this. In the first, participants focused discussion on their continued ability to care for themselves and their families. In the second, they encouraged us to view them over their life course, emphasising their past productivity. The strategies accord with 'identity control' theory (Burke, 2006). It posits that individuals manage their identities in response to threats by first aligning their behaviours with those in the desired identity standard, then over time, shifting the meanings of the behaviours held in the identity standard so that they accord with their current behaviour.

Continuing to care for oneself

Participants distanced their behaviours from those associated with their childlike possible self. Those not experiencing any significant age-related changes in their bodies did this by stressing their continued – or even increased – physical productivity. Highlighting their success in securing resources, they presented themselves as able to care for themselves and their families.

In this excerpt, Rabson singles out increasing work, wealth and providence as characteristic of his ageing experience. His older age is a period of 'growth', contrasting the period of decline he associates with others' ageing elsewhere in the interview:

> *I:* Now, what do you think has changed in your life in the last 20 years?
> *P:* Ah nothing...I haven't noticed the changes yet...I feel I am fine at the moment because I am able to work without any problems...[There is] no difference, and I can say I am feeling better now than before. Very much. You can see all these [points to his cotton garden and maize store]. I have done myself with my hands. I have also grown potatoes, pigeon peas...I am enjoying my growth...Even if the *alangizi* [Agricultural Advisor] comes today he would recommend my work in my fields. To me good life means being able to cultivate, children not lacking essential things. I thank God for that. (Rabson, male, 75)

Other participants were experiencing age-related declines in strength that made highly physical work more difficult. Nevertheless, they emphasised the continuation of their adult-compatible behaviours, distinguishing their 'prime' old age from the childlike 'very old' age, using a number of rhetorical strategies. Some stressed that they now worked harder to compensate for reduced strength:

> Aaa! I do the work while feeling pain. When I am able to move around I force myself to work...I am able to do my household chores. I also go to the garden and cultivate. For the waist and the eye, they have just started hurting...the arm pains a lot. (Loveness, female, late 70s)

Some qualified their reports of receiving care from their children with reports of the care they offered in return:

> Mainly it's when a person is very old that they would need someone to help them, but it should not be in everything...I am at the prime old person, I have not reached to be very old...My family benefit from me in many ways. One, they are happy they have a father and they do get support from me. Two, we do assist *each other* on the work which we undertake in this compound, [because] I act as the foreman. (Fiskani, male, 61)

Others stressed that although they could no longer perform some tasks, they continued to contribute to their self-care and household by performing other types of work:

> [Since last week] I have met the same problem of failing to walk, pain this side [pointing at his waist]...additional pain is from here [pointing at his chest]...I have worked a little. I was working while seated...I had some reeds for weaving and I was just processing them. (Charles, male, around 70)

Each of these narratives allowed participants to present themselves as people who, despite declining blood, are not unproductive, entirely dependent or unable to make any contribution to the care of others. In doing so, they managed the interviewer's and their own perceptions of their behaviour, realigning the meanings of their behaviour with those held as standard for the adult identity.

Emphasising past productivity

Other participants distanced themselves from the possible self by presenting current dependent behaviour within a discussion of 'usual' behaviour – that seen over a lifetime. Declines in strength and work were reported with reference to past self-reliance, productivity and care for dependants. Since the capital of a body is its ability to produce, in these narratives, the older body becomes a capital store, able to trade on past productivity. In the following example, Polly normalises her ageing experiences by focusing on care she has given. In doing so she presents the type of person she is: her underlying adult identity.

> I: You have talked about loss of strength in your body. How does that affect your life?
> P: I know it's because I am an old person...I used to carry a big bundle of firewood but nowadays I can't carry it, if I dare then I would feel pain in the head, neck, back, legs. Or cultivating, I can't do as I used to. In the past I was cultivating a large area before getting tired...I am not worried because I know I have stayed on this world for a long time...I am used to it now...every period has its own activities. I carry the bundle which I know I will manage... It can't be possible to go back and be a girl again. I was very powerful but I have shared it [her blood/power] with other people so I cannot be worried. (Polly, female, 60s)

In these narratives past productivity – care – represents the 'real' person. Ageing is something that happens to the body, leaving the adult 'inside' unchanged – akin to the 'ageing as a mask' theories of western gerontology (Featherstone and Hepworth, 1989). Receiving care in old age – that is, needing care and having care available – is a reflection of high past productivity, rather than a reflection of low present productivity. An individual is only without blood in old age *because* they have 'used up' so much of their finite store working hard. They had care available because they had cared for others. The adult identity is un-embodied as participants invite the interviewer to judge them on their past body-centred behaviour to indicate the type of person they are now. The meanings of the behaviour held in the adult identity standard are altered: to be an adult, one can have given everything. The strategy allowed older men and women to position the care they needed or received as evidence of the vitality and strength which they had invested in their relationships: they required care in later life *because* they were 'adults'.

Conclusion

This chapter highlights patterns in how older adults in rural Malawi made sense of receiving or not receiving care from their families in a series of conversations about ageing. In their narratives, the national and international construction of an 'African family' in which older adults become dependants that are (or at least were) cared for automatically appears to have little salience. Participants instead presented expectations of care in older age that were heavily dependent on notions of self-sufficiency and reciprocity, grounded in rural subsistence livelihoods.

The political assumption that older adults want care from their families doesn't accord with the more nuanced experiences of the older men and women in this study. Desire for familial care to be available was tempered by a desire to not need it. Inability to care for oneself was universally referenced as a bad old age. Participants' discussions centred on care as an embodied practice. As those by Obrist (Chapter Four) and De Klerk (Chapter Six), this chapter illustrates how incorporating the body and its meanings into the study of older age care in Africa can increase our understanding of how ageing and care are actually experienced. In Balaka, changing bodies had implications not only for older adults' activities and spaces, but for the self. For participants, inability to care presented a 'possible self' (Markus and Nurius, 1986) they resisted through identity work. Participants embarked on several discursive processes to reconcile receiving care with feeling that they were still 'adults' – participating members of the social world.

Extending consideration of older age care in Africa beyond questions of who receives care and how care is negotiated to questions of how giving and receiving care makes people feel, can enrich the political and academic conversation. Incorporating existing theories of identity into this discussion can lead to fuller understandings of older adults' experiences or expectations of care.

Notes

[1] Understood to include biological children and grandchildren, nieces, nephews and others if cared for when young.

[2] 'Bride price' paid to a wife's family. While common in the patrilineal north of Malawi it is not much practiced in the matrilineal south. Had Robertson paid labola in Balaka, where children belong to their mother's family, he would have 'owned' the children, so that on separation with their mother, they would have left with him and received his care daily.

[3] Elsewhere I have also used social psychological approaches to understanding the self to explore how older adults in Balaka based their identities on membership of the social group of 'adults'.

References

Aboderin, I, 2004, Modernisation and ageing theory revisited: Current explanations of recent developing world and historical western shifts in material family support for older people, *Ageing and Society* 24, 1, 29–50

Anglewicz, P, Adams, J, Obare, F, Kohler, H-P, Watkins, S, 2009, The Malawi Diffusion and Ideational Change Project 2004–06: data collection, data quality, and analysis of attrition, *Demographic Research* 20, 21, 503–40

Burke, P, 2006, Identity change, *Social Psychology Quarterly* 69, 1, 81–96

Burke, P, Reitzes, D, 1981, The link between identity and role performance, *Social Psychology Quarterly* 44, 2, 83–92

Burke, P, Tully, J, 1977, The measurement of role identity, *Social Forces* 55, 4, 881–97

Cattell, M, 1990, Models of old age among the Samia of Kenya: Family support of the elderly, *Journal of Cross-Cultural Gerontology* 5, 4, 375–94

Cattell, M, 2002, Holding up the sky: Gender, age and work among the Abaluyia of Kenya, in S Makoni, K Stroeken (eds) *Ageing in Africa: Sociolinguistic and anthropological approaches*, pp 155–76, Aldershot: Ashgate

Charmaz, K, 2006, *Constructing grounded theory: A practical guide through qualitative analysis*, London: SAGE Publications

Chintsanya, J, Chiwona-Karltun, L, Kaneka, B, Mandere, G, Jumali-Phiri, M, Pulcrino, R, Stloukal, L, 2010, *Current and expected trends in demographic composition and poverty characteristics of rural households*, Food and Agriculture Organisation of the United Nations report, Zomba: Department of Population Studies, Chancellor College University of Malawi

Comaroff, JL, Comaroff, J, 2001, On personhood: An anthropological perspective from Africa, *Social Identities* 7, 2, 267–83

Featherstone, M, Hepworth, M, 1989, Ageing and old age: Reflections on the postmodern life course, in B Bytheway, T Keil, P Allatt, A Bryman (eds) *Becoming and being old: Sociological approaches to later life*, pp 143–57, London: SAGE

Ferreira, M, 1999, Building and advancing African gerontology, *Southern African Journal of Gerontology* 8, 1, 1–3

Freeman, E, Coast, E, 2014, Sex in older age in rural Malawi, *Ageing and Society* 34, 7, 1118–41

Gilleard, C, Higgs, P, 2010, Aging without agency: Theorizing the fourth age, *Aging and Mental Health* 14, 2, 121–8

Guillette, E, 1992, *Finding the good life in the family and society: The Tswana aged of Botswana*, PhD thesis, Gainesville, FL: University of Florida

Luborsky, M, 1994, The cultural adversity of physical disability: Erosion of full adult personhood, *Journal of Aging Studies* 8, 3, 239–53

Markus, H, Nurius, P, 1986, Possible selves, *American Psychologist* 41, 9, 954–69

McCall, G, Simmons, J, 1966, *Identities and interactions*, New York: Free Press

NSO (National Statistical Office of Malawi), 2008, *Population and housing census data tables*, Zomba: National Statistical Office of Malawi, NSO

Peil, M, 1987, Studies of ageing in Africa, *Ageing and Society* 7, 4, 459–66

Schatz, E, Ogunmefun, C, 2007, Caring and contributing: The role of older women in rural South African multi-generational households in the HIV/AIDS era, *World Development* 35, 8, 1390–403

Schröder-Butterfill, E, Fithry, TS, 2014, Care dependence in old age: Preferences, practices and implications in two Indonesian communities, *Ageing and Society* 34, 3, 361–87

Sommer, BB, Sommer, R, 1991, *A practical guide to behavioral research: Tools and techniques*, 3rd edn, New York: Oxford University Press

Stets, J, Burke, P, 2000, Identity theory and social identity theory, *Social Psychology Quarterly* 63, 3, 224–37

Stroeken, K, 2002, From shrub to log: The ancestral dimension of elderhood among Sukuma in Tanzania, in S Makoni, K Stroeken (eds) *Ageing in Africa: Sociolinguistic and anthropological approaches*, pp 90–108, Aldershot: Ashgate

Twigg, J, 2006, *The body in health and social care*, Basingstoke: Palgrave Macmillan

UN (United Nations), 1982, Report of the World Assembly on Aging, Vienna, 26 July to 6 August 1982. New York: UN

UNDP (United Nations Development Programme), 2010, The real wealth of nations: Pathways to human development, in *Human development report 2010: 20th anniversary edition*, New York: UNDP

Van der Geest, S, 2002a, Respect and reciprocity: Care of elderly people in rural Ghana, *Journal of Cross–Cultural Gerontology* 17, 1, 3–31

Van der Geest, S, 2002b, The toilet: Dignity, privacy and care of elderly people in Kwahu, Ghana, in S Makoni, K Stroeken (eds) *Ageing in Africa: Sociolinguistic and anthropological approaches*, pp 227–44, Aldershot: Ashgate

WHO, 2001, *Definition of an older or elderly person*, World Health Organisation (WHO), http://www.who.int/healthinfo/survey/ageingdefnolder/en/

SIX

Making sense of neglect in northwest Tanzania

Josien de Klerk

Introduction

> When you are old
> And your back is bent
> And you have no child
> To whom will you belong?[1]
> *Saida Karoli*

These lyrics from a song by Saida Karoli, a popular Haya singer, convey the centrality of family and 'belonging to someone' in advanced old age, of having someone to rely on when physical strength is fading. As bodies age and change, older people's activities and abilities to engage in social relations change as well (Hastrup, 2005; Taylor, 2005). While physical decline is considered to be both normal and inevitable, older people's anticipation of the future makes changes to their physical strength a conscious concern.

In northwest Tanzania there are no formal care institutions, such as old-age homes, for older people. Former government employees receive a pension after retirement, but in rural villages these people are few, and mainly men. While solutions to the problem of old-age security are formulated by international advocacy organisations and local NGOs, at present the reality of old-age care in northwest Tanzania is that care for frail older people is mainly provided by the family. The ability of family members to provide this care has increasingly become insecure due to out-migration, adult death and economic deprivation.

At the same time, caring for dying children and orphaned grandchildren has played a large part in the lives of many older people, creating new challenges in intergenerational care relations. In this chapter the telling of stories about the neglect of people in their old age are analysed as observed during the course of a larger fieldwork project on experiences of ageing and care in the era of HIV/AIDS in a village in Kagera Region, northwest Tanzania. These stories illuminate older people's ideas about intergenerational care in the context of HIV/AIDS, and particularly their expectations for care in grandparent–adult grandchild relationships, which is here described as 'new constellations of care'. Although the introduction of antiretroviral medicines at the end of 2004 marked the beginning of a new era, described by older people as '*nafuu*' (relief), new long-term care demands also emerged. In households where members have multiple health concerns, long-term care involves constant negotiation over the distribution of scarce resources, including food, between household members, and often diverts attention away from the care needs of people in advanced old age.

Anxieties about being cared for in one's old age, which are caused both by the scarcity of resources and the uncertainty embedded in new constellations of care, are voiced through storytelling (see also Freeman, Chapter Five and Van der Geest, Chapter One). Elsewhere, I have discussed how storytelling has been analysed in terms of performance and empowerment (De Klerk, 2011). Fabian (2003) argues that storytelling is an action, one that is performative. Jackson (2002) further suggests that telling stories is a way for people to feel empowered: 'storytelling reworks and remodels subject–object relations in ways that subtly alter the balance between actor and acted upon, thus allowing us to feel that we actively participate in a world that for a moment seemed to discount, demean and disempower us' (2002, 16). Stories, then, are not sui generis, but emerge from and are located in a particular locality; their narratives and emotional logics are embedded in local relationships (De Klerk, 2011, 22).

In this case, during everyday visits with one another, older women discussed situations in which care was found wanting, which they talked about in terms of *roho mbaya* (a bad heart/soul) of caregivers, referring to an attitude of caregivers as well as their practice of caring. It could be that a caregiver just did the bare minimum but without treating an older person with respect, it could be that a caregiver did not even attend to an older person's basic needs, took valuable assets, such as property from the older person and, in the worst cases, physically abused the older person. Sometimes these stories were about a man living alone who did not receive appropriate care, but more typically they involved older women who were left with little or no care. I have chosen to capture these events with the term 'neglect', referring to older people's intended meaning; that some caregivers choose to not care or care only minimally.[2]

In analysing these stories it is important to realise that the values expressed in them are fluid. Values and the social practices they inform are shaped in the specific historical circumstances in which people are born and raised (Aldous, 1990, 573); they are subtly reshaped as people try to make sense of social changes in their older age. Generational roles, similarly, are shaped in everyday life, rather than being transmitted as an abstract set of values (Whyte et al, 2008).

This research shows that stories of neglect reveal personal concerns about the state of family care in the current era of HIV/AIDS and demonstrate older people's understandings of intergenerational relations in contemporary Kagera. They reflect hope that care in old age will materialise, but also the realisation that older people cannot necessarily expect to receive care.

Storytelling and events

Augustina, my co-researcher and I are sitting in the living room of Tibaigana's house, near the main road of the village. From the sofa, Tibaigana, in her mid-60s has a good view of the small path leading off the main road into the village and usually interrupts our daily chats with shouted greetings to villagers going up and down the road. A young man bikes past the house, carrying an old woman on the back of his bicycle. Tibaigana offers his name and explains that he went to fetch his grandmother from her natal home some 30 kilometres away, where she was beaten by her relatives.

These casual visits, which happened on a daily basis with Tibaigana and regularly with other older women and men, formed the core of the methodological approach in this research among older Haya, the main ethnic group in the Kagera region during 2003–04 (De Klerk, 2011). Understanding care as the outcome of relations that had been built over time, a longitudinal approach was employed, following 11 selected families over the course of a year. Information was collected through observing care events and collecting stories about these events. Different sides of each story were analysed, looking at what was at stake for the storyteller. This approach created a rich, nuanced view of the ambiguity of family care.

In 2005, 2008, and 2012 I returned to the village and visited the 11 families. Neglect emerged as a core theme. Of the 11 older people who had been followed initially, five had passed away. In three of those five deaths, my older interlocutors had deemed the care insufficient. In six of the 11 cases there were family conflicts around land and resources that had adverse effects on the provision of care. In two cases, adolescent granddaughters did provide daily care but protested against this obligation.

In the 2012 visit, I also interviewed nine older women and one man who were beneficiaries of the new cash transfer scheme and who had, over the course of their lives, raised orphaned grandchildren who had since started their own families. I attended social support group meetings facilitated by Kwa Wazee (for older people), a local NGO. Starting in 2004, Kwa Wazee has been providing a selected group of around 1,000 destitute older people with a monthly pension. Six of the 11 older people I had followed had become beneficiaries of the cash-transfer programme, just after I left the village in mid-2004.

In addition, the programme provided psycho-social support, and in later years added income-generating groups and a form of health promotion and insurance to their activities. As several of my interlocutors became members of the programme, I have been able to follow the effects of this new 'social institution' during subsequent visits. Finally, I spoke with ten adult grandchildren who had been raised by their grandparents, about caring for their old grandparents in their advanced old age. These interviews and data served as a broader backdrop for my analysis of stories, allowing me to assess the consequences of social interventions to counter neglect.

Experiences of ageing in northwest Tanzania

It is December 2003, in the middle of the cold rainy season. Augustina and I go to visit three elderly sisters who live together. The youngest, Maria, is 63 and disabled by a deformed leg. Maria and her son, who is also disabled, had no place to live after Maria's husband died, because he bequeathed his land to his other, healthy children born to his second wife. Veneta, 65, lost three of her four children to HIV between 1999 and 2002. She cared intensively for all of them and is now raising Matteo, her 8-year-old orphaned grandson. Sofia, 68, could not have children and her husband divorced her because of this. Not having had a son, the father of the three sisters bequeathed his land to them when he died at the age of 90. The house was left to Sofia as a form of old-age provision for a childless daughter. Sofia is strong: despite her age she fetches firewood and hauls water from the river that is some kilometres downhill. To obtain money for food and household expenses, the sisters work as casual labourers on other people's land.

Their main concern is losing their physical strength, as that will take away their only source of income. Today is such a day: because of the rainy season, everyone in the house is down with a cold. Young

Matteo is quite ill, coughing and lying on a mat in the grass-covered front room of the house. Veneta sits beside Matteo during the visit, but she herself has a headache and is shivering. Her two sisters are also coughing, and Maria is confined to bed. While we sit, Veneta attends to her ill grandson, checking his temperature, removing some clothes and watching over him. She repeatedly rests her head in her hands, in an expression of despair. They have shelter but no food, and no money to go to the hospital. There is no assistance from other family members.

As physical strength declines, the state of older people's relations becomes visible in the way care is organised. In the above situation, three older siblings care for each other and for a young grandchild, and they depend on their own strength to make a living. Biophysical changes such as ageing, have significant social consequences for daily life, social relations, identity and sense of self (Nettleton and Watson, 1998, 5). When older people in contemporary Kagera say '*sina nguvu*' (I have no strength), they refer to this uncertainty (see also Obrist, Chapter Four).

Illness has become a central aspect of the experience of ageing in Kagera – old age is no longer just linked to frailty, the long process of mental and physical decline but also to ill-health (Livingston, 2003). Older people are more susceptible to pneumonia and malaria, especially in the cold nights that accompany the rainy seasons. Many older people suffer from chronic illnesses such as high blood pressure, diabetes and heart problems, and often have multiple other health problems, such as difficulty walking due to pain, intestinal pain, toothaches, hearing problems and cataracts. Obrist (Chapter Four) refers to these illness episodes as 'critical health moments' in which older people actively become aware of their bodies.

In addition to suffering from age-related vulnerabilities and illnesses, the bodies of many older women were taxed by years of intensive palliative caregiving, performed before antiretroviral medicines became available. Caring for a dying patient involves fetching firewood to cook specific foods, washing a patient, spoon-feeding, sitting vigil at night, accompanying a patient to the outside toilet and washing soiled sheets in the river. It also involves psychological distress, and many caregivers reported not being able to sleep at night because of worries and grief (Ssengonzi, 2007; De Klerk, 2011; Wright et al, 2012). These confrontations with tired bodies and loss shaped how older people imagine their old age and the presence of others to provide care.

Concerns over frailty are visible in the subtle ways local terms for advanced old age are used. Advanced age is defined on the basis of social age, such as having grandchildren and physical capacity, with a difference made between older people who have strength (*mkaile* in vernacular) and those who don't. Older people without strength are called *mkaikuru* (female) and *mgurusi* (male). The *ability* of the ageing body is now seen as a central part of wellbeing; older people feel compelled to stay active for as long as possible (Sagner, 2002; Bohman et al, 2007; see also Freeman, Chapter Five).

Actual care arrangements in old age and how these were perceived, need to be situated in the 'historical times' in which different generations of older people grew up and had children (see also Hoffman, Chapter Seven). Sibling-to-sibling care, as we see in the situation of Veneta, Maria and Sofia, has historical roots; often epidemiological, or political-economic upheavals (De Klerk, 2011; Seeley, 2014). One such epidemiological upheaval was a widespread epidemic of venereal disease in the first half of the previous century which has influenced birth-rates and caused high levels of infertility and divorce (Larsson, 1991; Stevens, 1991). For the historical generation that grew up during this period the presence of children to provide care in old age was never a certainty, and this shaped ideas among this historical generation about how to prepare for old age.

The generation of their children, who was able to have (many) children in the second half of the previous century, was ageing when the AIDS-epidemic hit the region from the mid-1980s onwards. Rising birth rates and rapid population growth in the second half of the century had created an expectation among this historical generation that the children who survived childhood would live and care for them in old age. Losing multiple family members to AIDS, not only young adult children but also often partners, siblings and in-laws who all formed part of the broader family care circle, was a devastating shock, forcing them to adjust their expectations for older age care (see De Klerk, 2011).

By 2012, having reached advanced old age and having raised many orphaned grandchildren into adulthood, many had transferred their expectations for care to their adult grandchildren, even though this created a predicament for these adult grandchildren: how to combine the care for an elderly person with the need to start their own lives.

The delivery of care in Kagera then is, in essence, about belonging and about circumstance: it depends on who is present at a certain moment in time (see also Freeman, Chapter Five), who is able to care and what the physical condition of the older person is. Although care arrangements are fluid, a constant is that the primary caregivers for elderly people are those with whom an older person has built a relationship of intimacy and closeness over time (see also Whyte and

Whyte, 2004). Equally so, expectations of care are also fluid and reflect personal biographies and historical events particular to the region.

In the following sections, I present the stories that emerged around one case of neglect during my main fieldwork in 2003/4 (see also De Klerk, 2011),[3] and examine how other older people came to terms with the neglect through storytelling. The case highlights how care is the outcome of shared lives (Whyte and Whyte, 2004) and existing conflicts and closeness, but also of chance. This is the story of Tophista, the woman on the back of the bicycle, from the moment her grandson brought her to the village until her death some months later.

When the body turns frail: Tophista's loss of care in advanced old age

Tophista was 86, frail and bedridden when we met her for the first time. She was being cared for by the young wife of one of her grandsons, who was struggling to make ends meet. Staying with adult grandchildren was not how Tophista had envisioned her old age. She had been wealthy, lived in the regional capital Bukoba, and inherited land from her father and her husband. After her husband died and her only son inherited the house, she remained there, living with him, which was a common arrangement for many elderly widows. But in 2000 her son died from AIDS, following his wife. His death rendered her suddenly childless at an already advanced old age. This situation demanded the establishment of new relations of care.

Initially, Tophista remained in her former marital home, which was now inherited by her youngest grandson, Laurent. He had promised his father to take care of his grandmother, but, being only 19 at this time, and unmarried, he called his sister, asking whether they could move in with her and her children and to provide the intimate daily care Tophista needed. Fed up with the children running through the land and ruining the crops, Tophista and her granddaughter had a fall out. When Laurent chose his sister's side, Tophista decided to move to her natal home, 30 kilometres away, to live with her siblings.

The decisions she made around this move created further discord in the family. Not planning to ever come back, and in order to have money for her everyday expenses, she sold the land with the family graves, which she had inherited from her husband. Infuriated, her brother-in-law, 87-year-old Vedasto, intervened and asked his son to buy the land back. Tophista also distributed the money from the land sale unevenly; she decided to not give Laurent anything and gave money to only two of her 13 grandchildren, strengthening the relations she trusted most, but alienating others. 'I sold one *shamba* [plot of land] to pay the bride price of my grandson…I sold three *shamba*s to care for myself as I am sick and have no strength.'

Unfortunately, the decision to move to her natal home backfired. Hearing that she was being beaten and neglected there, one of her grandsons wanted to bring her back to the village. Vedasto, the family patriarch, advised against it, as he envisioned more and more problems emerging because this particular grandson had lost most of the money Tophista had given him and was not able to take care of her himself. Despite these warnings, the grandson moved Tophista back to his home, where we first met her. Vedasto's warnings quickly became reality: the grandson left the village in search of work and his young wife had to return Tophista to Laurent's house, where she continued to reside until her death in May 2004.

Newly married, Laurent assigned his wife the everyday care of his grandmother, but with ambivalence: 'This is because of my good heart – any other person would not have done so, as she [Tophista] does not love me and never gave me anything.' Tophista felt uncomfortable living there. Visiting her one day, she pointed at the banana plantation around her and said:

> This is the *shamba* which was mine and which I sold. Now nobody cares for me. All are blaming me, that is why I sold my *shamba*. But I sold it when I decided to go [to my natal home], thinking I would stay there. But now nobody is caring for me, not even giving me a single cent of money. While before I was rich, giving things to people. *Ninshaba owonaimile nimanya akebwa* [Haya proverb: now I am asking something of the one I once refused, hoping he has forgotten that I once refused].

Over the course of the following months, Tophista's situation kept deteriorating: she became confused, and her behaviour changed every time she saw us. She would scratch herself, moan and shiver, and often almost fell to the floor. She started to wolf down food and tea, her body smelled of urine, and her feet were infested with jiggers (chigoe fleas) and her skin was dry. She felt uncared for, and tried to run away and to commit suicide with a *panga* (a large cutting knife). In the end Laurent had to lock her in a room when he and his wife were working on the land. She died there a few months later.

Talking neglect

Over the months we followed Tophista's life, we collected stories that reflected different perceptions about and attitudes towards care among older people in the village. By telling stories, family members and neighbours attempted to make sense of the neglect they were witnessing. Tophista's lack of care served as an event that made visible the cracks in family care that everyone knew existed. In the following section, I discuss Tophista's neglect from three points of view as found in these stories:

- how older people are supposed to build relations of care for themselves in this era;
- how older people feel that they can keep some control over their care;
- how older people relate neglect to the structural conditions in which care is to take place in contemporary Kagera.

Care as the outcome of closeness

As soon as Tophista started displaying to us physical signs of neglect – showing us her feet infested with jiggers and scratching at her dry skin – Augustina, who was not only a co-researcher but also a Haya woman and a nurse – became infuriated. She started to cook for Tophista and blamed the caregivers for not showing *huruma* (compassion), a central value of close relations in Kagera. Compassion, according to older people, was slowly disappearing in the younger generation; the older women we spoke with often became indignant, giving many examples of adults not showing compassion when caring for their elderly parents. The lack of compassion, according to older people, was found in everyday aspects of life: a bereaved mother going to the market *during* her child's funeral, a son stealing the land deed from his blind father, a fat woman coming to visit from town while her father was living in a dilapidated house. Older people argued that, no matter what the parent had or had not done, compassion was part of care.

A second narrative in the stories told about Tophista's situation contradicted this premise of unconditional compassion: care in advanced old age was the outcome of relations that had been built in a good manner over the course of a lifetime. Tophista had only invested financially in the two grandsons she trusted, and this was seen as a mistake. Doing so made perfect sense to Tophista, as she did not expect to ever go back to her former marital home and she decided to strengthen the relationship with the two grandsons she had been close to all along. From the perspective of her family and her neighbours, however, the discord she created did not befit an old person. Tophista herself acknowledged this when she spoke of being blamed and used a proverb to ask for forgiveness. Despite recognising the lack of compassion in Laurent's behaviour, through storytelling neighbours constructed a moral world in which they could understand neglect as the outcome of Tophista's bad judgement.

Caregiving is a set of interactions as well as a process that unfolds over the course of a relationship (Mol, 2008). While everyday care for older women – cooking; fetching water and firewood; and assistance with bathing, washing clothes and visiting the toilet – could be done by adolescent granddaughters, daughters-in-law, or a hired house girl, care for older women in times of illness was almost always performed by specific relatives, usually a daughter or a sister. Intimate 'loving' care, given when someone is ill, weak, or very old, is an indication of a good relationship that has been built over a lifetime. Seeley et al (2009) call this 'linked lives'. Older people call this 'leaning on', or being 'carried on the back', phrases that describe how close relatives compensate for the loss of physical strength (see Sagner, 2002).

Kaijage (1997) argues that when the HIV/AIDS epidemic reached its peak in 1987 in the Kagera region, the increasing nuclearisation of the family meant that the extended family system of care had ceased to function. In the past, brothers of a deceased man were supposed to provide for ill and ageing widows and orphans in the deceased's home, in order to safeguard any male orphan's claim to his father's land and provide a safety net for the clan's female members (Kaijage, 1997). This 'ideal' system has indeed disappeared, although one has to question whether it ever existed in reality. Bonds of affection, mostly formed in the natal home, and the increase in more formalised care through the many mutual support groups, shape care in advanced old age, rather than entitlements in a marital home. The increased precariousness of care now shapes older women's experiences of physical ageing and the way the older body is read in the village.

The quality of care in advanced old age becomes visible in the well-tended body, thus making the elderly body a reflection of the state of family relations. A well-nurtured and clean body was seen as indicative of an older person's health and wellbeing (see also Weiss, 1997, 343). Through appearance, elderly people are able to show who cares for them, which reflects positively on their caregivers. In this sense the temporal aspect of relational care is important: as older people grow older and more dependent, they increasingly need to draw upon care relations to ensure their dignity. Dignity is an expression of good relations, manifested in a nicely dressed body, shining skin, being well fed, and surrounded by grandchildren. Zulia, in her mid-80s, who lost all five of her children, proudly pointed to her adult grandson, whom she raised and with whom she now lives, and at her skin when I asked her about care. Smelling nicely of body lotion, she said, smiling: 'You see, I am shining!'

To subtly remind caregivers of their presence, some older women like Tophista would talk about feeling weak and having pain, or express self-pity (see also Pype, Chapter Two). A central social value in Haya society is that of *enclosure*, which is the need to conceal anything that could relay information about a household and hence affect its social standing. This value is visible in all aspects of life, including wrapping gifts, disclosing one's whereabouts and eating: Haya will not eat with the door open or in other people's houses, as food is indicative of socioeconomic status (Weiss, 1996), and can be used to do harm through poisoning. When Tophista started to wolf down food in front of us and later accepted tea in Tibaigana's house, gulping down the hot liquid, she was directly accusing her caregivers of not caring for her. When she showed us her feet, and complained of dry skin and scratched herself, she was trying to shame her caregivers to caring for her. Though older people in advanced old age were unable to use their physical strength they still used their physical appearance to say something about the quality of their care.

Explicit complaints were, however, often ascribed to '*tamaa*', an unrealistic desire. In one roadside conversation about the life stage of old age, a woman said:

> They are just complaining. The problem is if someone is old, even the mind decreases. Maybe what he is expecting the child to do for him is not what the child is doing. So the old person complains even though he is being cared for. But he is not satisfied. It is not according to his expectation, which is more than the *uwezo* [means, wealth] of the child.

This criticism stemmed from the value of enclosure: older people who were respected were those who did not complain, those who were not enforcing care by shaming relatives.

Stories about Tophista linked her bodily displays explicitly to shame, but not the shame of her caregivers. As Tophista was neglected by a young person to whom she had never given anything, she herself was blamed for not building her relationships better. By understanding neglect in these terms, older people around her created a narrative that justified her neglect. The moral lesson was clear: relationships must be carefully built and maintained throughout one's life, and possessions should never be squandered. This is the subject of the next section.

Preparing for old age: older people's self-responsibility

A common narrative among older people in the village was that people had to prepare for old age. As events began to rapidly unfold in Tophista's life, we started to visit more often. Tibaigana, to whom we confided our frustration over Tophista's lack of care, commented:

> You know that if you do not keep any property for yourself in later life, you will suffer when you become old. If she could have kept a *shamba* or a house or other things, she could have been cared for, because those who would care for her would be able to get food from the *shamba*. But no one is going to care for you when they also have to do casual labour for food and money for expenses. It is not easy to get help.

Older people see land as a durable asset, contrary to the volatility of money. Land generates food, for both income and subsistence, and has a social value; by burying their dead on clan land next to the house, Haya ensure generational continuity on the land. This practice connects generations of ancestors to living relatives. By selling land with graves on it, Tophista not only created discord in her family but, what is more important, lost the possibility of endowing land. Endowing is a Haya social practice whereby one generation transfers authority to the next and in that process glues generations together through the inheritance of valuable land. Providing materially for your children (and nowadays also orphaned grandchildren) is a central value of intergenerational relations; endowing is expected to lead to care, but if not done properly might lead to neglect.

Expectations of care are influenced by norms derived from the *ekibanja* system, the system of landholding and sharing that informs the spatial settlement of families and structures inheritance between generations. Gender is an important factor that determines how one is able to provide. In the past, an older widowed woman was not allowed to inherit, and her husband's family was supposed to provide care in her advanced old age. Today, many widowed women do have some access to the use of land, but unless they buy land themselves, their position is far more insecure than that of older men who have always been allowed to inherit. There are many single women who live on small pieces of land or who have no land at all; they live off their own casual labour, just getting by, until their strength fails. In this context, when Tophista, who was once wealthy and inherited land, sold her land, this was seen as reckless behaviour.

Endowing can also build new relations of care with others, including non-kin: land can be promised as inheritance in return for care. This practice of endowing as a strategy to consolidate new relations of care has a history among older Haya. As a result of the epidemic of venereal disease in the first half of the last century, many women who were in their 80s in early 2000 – like Tophista – had very few children or were barren. The majority of these women, nonetheless, had found ways to obtain land: through inheritance from their fathers or through buying land. Land was seen as a durable investment because of its potential to bind children and non-kin. A woman of 86, who had lost all three children to AIDS and was now living with an older brother, voiced this poignantly: 'I went to the city where I had these children [through commercial sex work]. I came back after seven years and bought land. But they died and I sold the land, I did not see the point of keeping it any more.' The pension initiated by Kwa Wazee for destitute older people described earlier is seen as a similar kind of asset: ensured of a regular income until their death, older people employ that income as a durable asset and use it to 'buy' care from non-kin.

The focus on land in older people's stories not only highlights its potential to secure care, but also its potential to be the centre of generational clashes. The death of adults who left behind young (male) children, not yet able to farm but still entitled to the land of their fathers, increased conflicts over land. Many grandparents tried to safeguard land for their orphaned grandchildren from relatives trying to claim the land, starting court cases and writing wills. Then there were many older people ageing without land, or with only small plots after having to sell land to cover costs of caregiving and funerals. Even though many older people tried to prepare themselves for old age, many were unable to hold on to that most valuable asset, land.

Despite this, preparing for old age by retaining land, a house and assets remains one of the ways in which older people try to manage the uncertainties of declining bodily strength. Observing Tophista's mental confusion and irate behaviour, older people did not attribute such things to senescence but rather interpreted them as a consequence of shame from losing all her wealth and possessions, from not being responsible for herself.

Beyond shame: neglect as a consequence of new constellations of care

The village chairman related Tophista's lack of care to the young age of her primary caregiver. Laurent was only 21 and newly married. Tophista was 86, mentally confused and incontinent. She did not want to eat standard Haya food: cooked bananas, which is all the young new wife was able to give her. Caring for her was hard work, and the life stage of the young newly married couple, trying to start their lives together, did not mesh well with the care demands of advanced old age. Acknowledging this, the chairman compared the care for several older women in the village at that time:

> If you look at Nuria (86): she is *leaning on* her brother (83). If he hears that his wife does not take good care of her, he will make trouble. And my mother (88), same story: when she was young, she did not inherit land. It was all given to a sister. When that sister aged and needed care, my mother did not hold a grudge, she cared for her. They were both acting as mature people.

Laurent, who was young, economically broke, and holding a grudge against his grandmother, was in no position to care properly. The chairman, seeing this type of problem emerging more frequently, did not blame Laurent as such but linked the lack of care to the increasing problem of the lack of presence of those who can provide care.

Care is related to decision-making power in families. Laurent was young but he was running his own household, and his wife had to follow his lead when caring for Tophista. When older women discussed situations where care was found wanting, they almost always associated the care provided with the level of decision-making power of caregivers in the broader family (see Janzen, 1978). Close bonds do not necessarily have to exist between the older person and the primary caregiver; relations of care are often triangular relations, in which having a close relationship with a decision maker can also result in care. Nuria, a childless, witty and cheerful old woman, who lived with her older brother and his wife, was not close with her sister-in-law. Her sister-in-law cared for her, but only because her husband told her to do so. When Nuria fell ill in 2004, at the age of 86, her sisters came from neighbouring villages and together nursed her back to health. In 2005, when her brother fell seriously ill, I visited her. She spoke about the past year, becoming pensive, and she pointed to the back room where her brother was confined to bed, saying: 'I just pray to die first. If he dies I will die soon too'. She indeed died three months after his death. While Nuria's close relationship with the decision maker ensured that she received care, Tophista's conflict with Vedasto, the person who had the power in her family, led to her neglect. These examples show that care is an outcome of broader kinship biographies (Dilger, 2010); similarly, discussions of Tophista's neglect were discussions about the dissolution of her family. Indeed, in 2012, Laurent and his wife had separated, following the death of their baby, and Laurent had left the village.

With the maturing of the HIV/AIDS epidemic, and of the many orphaned grandchildren, the question of who will care for their elderly grandmothers has become urgent. In 2012, during follow-up research, most of the older women in their 60s and 70s who had been caring for dying patients and raising small children in 2003/4, had reached advanced old age. Many of them were still providing care, but also increasingly needed care themselves. Seeing their grandchildren as their children, they held the same expectations, but also realised that such relations were less certain; grandchildren married or moved out of the region to obtain an education. Grandchildren themselves were torn between the responsibility they felt towards their grandmothers and their need to start their own lives. Many grandchildren had very warm, close relationships with their grandmothers, unlike the relationship between Tophista and Laurent. In those cases, a surviving child or an adult grandchild would send an adolescent daughter to live with the elderly grandmother, keep her company, and do everyday chores, but there were also cases like that of Tophista where no one was present to provide care.

During fieldwork in 2003/4, similar arrangements were found, and although such 'new constellations of care' were not as widespread it does suggest that care arrangements have long been both uncertain and diverse in Kagera. In 2003/4, many older women who had few or no children were reaching advanced old age; some lived with siblings back in their natal homes, others lived with non-kin, or moved between places (see also Pype, Chapter Two).

Older people with children made it clear that they did not think it was obligatory (*lazima*) for their children to care for them; care was something they hoped for, but they also fully understood the difficult economic predicaments faced by many adults. Adult children, when they are able, support their parents by buying everyday necessities like kerosene, cooking oil, salt and soap, paying for medical expenses, and providing cash and luxury items such as televisions, mobile phones and video players. Older people were well aware of the challenges their adult children were facing in providing care for them, and as long as their children visited regularly and assisted a bit, they were never criticised.

Non-kin care

As a result of the uncertainty of old-age care and the enormous costs of regular funerals different mechanisms emerged in the village. The most important one was the mutual support group. In 2003/4, these groups mainly comprised burial associations, religious groups and women's groups (Dercon et al, 2006); there had been a mushrooming of these groups before 2000 when many people were dying from HIV/AIDS and neighbourly support during funerals (providing food and water for funeral guests, fetching firewood, digging graves) was rapidly decreasing. When a close relative of one of the group's members died, the members of the group all paid a defined contribution. Older people said that it was imperative to be a member of such a group, and some even worked to earn money to pay the contribution (De Klerk, 2011). While belonging to such groups prevented older people from having to sell valuable land, other mechanisms to obtain money, such as advance selling of the coffee harvest for the coming season or taking out loans with land as collateral, contributed to further deprivation.

In 2004, recognising the increasing number of older people living in difficult circumstances, Kwa Wazee started a pilot cash-transfer programme. Destitute older people without care, impoverished grandmothers raising grandchildren, and single older women and men without care, qualified. A monthly stipend was accompanied by participation in mutual support groups. A recent evaluation showed that older people who were part of the programme more often engaged in loans and transactions, including within their families (Hofmann and Heslop, 2014). The organisation quickly realised, however, that the increasing availability of money did not alleviate the problems in care provision. When one of my informants, a disabled woman of 68, died from neglect, a new kind of health scheme was organised: when one of the group members falls ill, other group members go and take over household duties, accompany the sick member to the hospital, and donate food and firewood. This involvement of non-kin in care also functions as a moral reminder to family members to provide care.

Looking 'sideways', as Vaughan (1983) suggests, at these non-kin institutions can illuminate hidden transactions in family care. In Kagera, the existence of and need for non-kin institutions confirm the limits of land endowment as a practice to bind care relations and reveal the insecurity of kin-based care. Older people all described the health support group as the most important support they received, even though it only applied to short illness events.

How do these interventions in family care reframe experiences of physical ageing? Veneta, Maria and Sofia became members of the NGO pension programme in 2004. With this assistance, they have been able to school their grandchild Matteo, who is now 16 and still living with his grandmother and great aunts, helping them in the household. Sofia has since passed away and while Veneta and Maria still work on their land, they no longer have to work as casual labourers to earn money for food and daily expenses. Other older women involved in a health and exercise programme also provided by the NGO, state that they are able to do more in the house and are able to socialise because they can walk short distances again. Pension money was used for everyday necessities but also to hire labour, which allowed older people to rest their bodies (Hofmann and Heslop, 2014). A physical exercise programme to mobilise the very old, improved mobility and decreased dependence. This had vastly improved the relations with care providers.

Advice on eating particular nutritious foods, such as spinach, avocados and fruits, and an intervention to clean drinking water, through SODIS, Solar Water Disinfection,[4] had led to improved feelings of strength and to decreased conflicts over household tasks between older people and their grandchildren. By providing a platform where illness and body pains can be discussed, such health programmes also illuminate how much bodily conditions shape the everyday activities of older people. The statement '*sina nguvu*' (I have no strength) is not only a metaphor to discuss the experience of ageing in rapidly changing configurations of care, it is also very much a statement that foreshadows the physical experience of ageing in contemporary Kagera.

Conclusion

Older people, through telling stories about neglect, make sense of their anxiety regarding the essential insecurity embedded in the social relations in contemporary Kagera. The need to remain physically strong and the social emphasis on self-responsibility in arranging old-age care make older women acutely aware of their ageing bodies and their changing abilities.

The case of Tophista, a dependent elderly woman, demonstrates how different people – an older neighbour, the family patriarch and the village chairman – differently interpreted her neglect, each from their own perspective. This case shows how much older people and those around them construct their old age, and the care that they receive in that phase, as a period of time for which they are responsible themselves. In doing so, older people reinforce generational norms of compassion, enclosure and endowment – values that they feel have been to some extent lost among today's young people. But at the same time, the attribution of blame intersects with a pragmatic realisation that life for young people is difficult and that one can hope for but not expect care. Pragmatism also shows in the joining of mutual support groups, the main constellation of care outside of kin networks. Because enclosure is such a central cultural value, in some cases the involvement of non-kin in care functions as a moral reminder to family.

Care as a result of its very close, interpersonal nature, poses questions of what good care entails and what is seen as neglect. Caregiving takes place in a local moral world (Kleinman, 2006), one that is not fixed but constantly reinvented, through stories and observations about care, through generational references to a shared past, and through pragmatic observations of the contemporary reality of care. In this sense, expectations for care constantly shift as society shifts. Grandmothers start to hope for care from young adult grandchildren, because grandparent–grandchildren households have become a normal social reality. The life-stage and maturity of these grandchildren might mean that practices of caregiving might change: intimate care might be outsourced to non-kin, and new definitions of 'kin' might emerge as same-generation health support groups of older people increasingly become a resource for older people needing care.

Notes

[1] These lines from a popular Haya song were quoted to me by an 86-year-old, childless woman, who was dependent on her younger brother. She used it to discuss issues of respect and future care for women without children. When her brother died in 2005, she died only a few months later.

[2] In doing so I am aware that subtle meanings often get lost in a translation and that the connotation of neglect in English might differ slightly from the broader meaning it is assigned in this chapter.

[3] This chapter is based on ideas first worked out in my dissertation titled *Being old in times of AIDS: Aging, caring and relating in northwest Tanzania* (De Klerk, 2011). Follow-up research in 2012 with the same families strengthened the initial analysis in the dissertation and traced developments in care over time.

[4] This technique uses cleaned transparent PET bottles. If such a bottle is filled with water and placed in the morning sun and exposed for at least six hours, the majority of parasites causing intestinal problems are killed and the water becomes safe for consumption. This technique was implemented among elderly support group members registered with Kwa Wazee.

Acknowledgements

The author wishes to thank Marleen de Witte, Eileen Moyer, Marian Burchardt, Erin Martineau and Sjaak van der Geest for comments on earlier drafts of this chapter.

References

Aldous, J, 1990, Family development and the life course: Two perspectives on family change, *Journal of Marriage and the Family* 52, 3, 571–83

Bohman, D, Vasuthevan, S, Van Wyk, N, Ekman, S, 2007, We clean our houses, prepare for weddings and go to funerals: Daily lives of elderly Africans in Majaneng, South Africa, *Journal of Cross-Cultural Gerontology* 22, 323–37

De Klerk, J, 2011, *Being old in times of AIDS: Aging, caring and relating in northwest Tanzania*. Leiden: Africa Studies Centre

Dercon, S, De Weerdt, J, Bold, T, Pankhurst, A, 2006, Group-based funeral insurance in Ethiopia and Tanzania, *World Development* 34, 4, 685–703

Dilger, H, 2010, My relatives are running away from me! Kinship and care in the wake of structural adjustment, privatisation and HIV/AIDS in Tanzania, in H Dilger, U Luig (eds) *Morality, hope and grief: Anthropologies of AIDS in Africa*, pp 102–24, New York: Berghahn Books

Fabian, J, 2003, Forgetful remembering: A colonial life in the Congo, *Africa*, 73, 4, 489–504

Hastrup, K, 2005, *A passage to anthropology: Between experience and theory*, New York: Routledge

Hofmann, S, Heslop, M, 2014, *Towards universal pensions in Tanzania: Evidence on opportunities and challenges from a remote area, Ngenge Ward, Kagera*, London: HelpAge International Report

Jackson, M, 2002, *The politics of storytelling: Violence, transgression and intersubjectivity*, Copenhagen: Museum Tusculanum Press

Janzen, J, 1978, *The quest for therapy: Medical pluralism in lower Zaire*, Berkeley, CA: University of California Press

Kaijage, F, 1997, Social exclusion and the social history of disease: The impact of HIV/AIDS and the changing concept of the family in northwestern Tanzania, in S McGrath, C Jedrej, K Kind, J Thompson (eds) *Rethinking African history*, pp 331–56, University of Edinburgh: Centre of African Studies

Kleinman, A, 2006, *What really matters: Living a moral life amidst uncertainty and danger*, Oxford: Oxford University Press

Larsson, B, 1991, *Conversion to greater freedom? Women, church and social change in northwestern Tanzania under colonial rule*, Uppsala: Almqvist and Wiksell

Livingston, J, 2003, Reconfiguring old age: Elderly women and concerns over care in southeastern Botswana, *Medical Anthropology* 22, 3, 205–31

Mol, A, 2008, *The logic of care: Health and the problem of patient choice*, New York: Routledge

Nettleton, S, Watson, J, 1998, *The body in everyday life*, London: Routledge

Sagner, A, 2002, Identity management and old age construction among Xhosa-speakers in urban South Africa: Complaint discourse revisited, in S Makoni, K Stroeken (eds) *Ageing in Africa: Socio-cultural and linguistic approaches*, pp 43–66, Aldershot: Ashgate Publishing Limited

Seeley, J, 2014, *HIV and East Africa: Thirty years in the shadow of an epidemic*, New York: Routledge

Seeley, J, Wolff, B, Kabunga, E, Tumwekwase, G, Grosskurth, H, 2009, This is where we buried our sons: People of advanced old age coping with the impact of the AIDS epidemic in a resource-poor setting in rural Uganda, *Ageing and Society* 29, 115–34

Ssengonzi, R, 2007, The plight of older persons as caregivers to people infected/affected by HIV/AIDS: Evidence from Uganda, *Journal of Cross-Cultural Gerontology* 22, 4, 339–53

Stevens, L, 1991, Religious change in a Haya village, *Journal of Religion in Africa* 21, 1, 2–25

Taylor, J, 2005, Surfacing the body interior, *Annual Review of Anthropology* 34, 741–56

Vaughan, M, 1983, Which family? Problems in the reconstruction of the history of the family as an economic and cultural unit, *The Journal of African History* 24, 2, 275–83

Weiss, B, 1996, *The making and unmaking of the Haya lived world: Consumption, commoditization, and everyday practice*, Durham, NC: Duke University Press

Weiss, B, 1997, Northwestern Tanzania on a single shilling: Sociality, embodiment, valuation, *Cultural Anthropology* 12, 3, 335–61

Whyte, S, Whyte, M, 2004, Children's children: Time and relatedness in Eastern Uganda, *Africa* 74, 1, 76–94

Whyte, S, Alber, E, Van der Geest, S, 2008, Generational connections and conflicts in Africa: An introduction, in E Alber, S van der Geest, S Whyte (eds) *Generations in Africa: Connection and conflicts*, pp 1–26, Berlin: LIT Verlag

Wright, S, Zalwango, F, Seeley, J, Mugisha, J, Scholten, F, 2012, Despondency among HIV-positive older men and women in Uganda, *Cross-Cultural Gerontology* 27, 4, 319–33

SEVEN

Negotiating care for older people in South Africa: between the ideal and the pragmatics

Jaco Hoffman

Introduction

In this chapter we position ourselves at the intersection of current socio-economic and epidemiological trends with population ageing but also at the interface of care and the family. Care[1] here refers to a wide continuum of exchanges by individuals to one another, both tangible and intangible (see Kahn and Antonucci, 1980). The capacity of family networks to care for both older as well as younger dependants is severely limited by socio-economic factors but also by the impact of pandemics such as HIV/AIDS. This is specifically the case, for example, in Sub-Saharan Africa (SSA), where caregiving is negotiated within constrained societal development with family poverty a common phenomenon, which is further exacerbated by the AIDS pandemic in particular. HIV/AIDS-infected people in South Africa number around 6 million with an estimated 1.2 million children orphaned by AIDS. Approximately 60 per cent of these orphans live in grandparent-headed multi-generational families with particularly grandmothers acting as surrogate parents. These grandmothers often also simultaneously care for HIV-positive adult and/or unemployed children. Some academic, policy and programmatic concern, particularly in the context of HIV/ AIDS, has focused on the economic and social costs of care provided *by* older to younger generations, but the attention focused on the other part of the configuration – the question of care *for* older persons – is negligible. The following questions call for answers: Who will care for these older carers when they are in need of social and health care? How will the experiential aspects of the current intergenerational support and the understanding of such support norms relate to future expectations of generational support for older generations?

Through a generational sequential[2] analysis based on 58 narratives from 20 Nguni-speaking multi-generational networks conducted over the period of two years in the city of Emalahleni, Mpumalanga (South Africa), this chapter sets out to explore expectations for the future care of older people where there is currently mainly downward support by older generations for younger generations. It further endeavours to establish how these expectations impact on intergenerational dynamics. The up to five generations interviewed are broadly located in roughly three historically distinctive periods ranging from the so-called 'disempowered' Apartheid older/oldest generations (G1/G2) through the 'struggle' generations (G2/G3 – middle generations) to the youngest generations – the grandchildren (G3) and great-grandchildren (G4/G5) from the post-Apartheid era.

These identified historical markers are widely acknowledged as turning points in the political, social and economic life of South Africans (Ramphele, 1993). Combined, they cover the entire Apartheid era as well as the immediate post-Apartheid period. It is important to note the period in which the participants in this research lived the largest part of their formative years are used to determine the cohorts within which they are located.

Older submissive-resilient Apartheid generations

The participants from this era are aged between 64 to 94 years, having been born between 1915 and 1944. This era is characterised by passive resistance against Apartheid. Naturally the oldest generations in this study fall in this period. They had lived through Apartheid – they had experienced through the course of their lives the cumulative effects of marginalisation and many disadvantages as well as losses (Ferreira, 2004b).

The struggle generations

The period between the Sharpeville massacre (1960) and events leading up to the democratic elections in 1994 can be characterised by the armed struggle against Apartheid. Oliver Tambo and Nelson Mandela hailed the black youth as the *young lions* who took over as the shock troops of the revolution while they and other ageing black leaders were in exile and locked away in prison.

This period in the history of South Africa was marked by the events of 21 March 1960 when 69 people were killed in what became known as the Sharpeville massacre. A storm of international protest followed, including sympathetic demonstrations in many countries and condemnation by the United Nations. On 1 April 1960 the United Nations Security Council passed Resolution 134 whereupon South Africa found itself increasingly isolated from the international community. On home soil the Sharpeville massacre also led to the banning of the Pan Africanist Congress (PAC) and the African National Congress (ANC) which was one of the catalysts for a shift from passive resistance to armed resistance by these organisations. This also led to the establishment of Poqo, the military wing of the PAC, and Umkhonto we Sizwe, the military wing of the ANC.

Another significant marker during this period was the Soweto student uprising on 16 June 1976 when 23 people were killed on the first day, including several black teenagers. The riots continued and resulted in the deaths of 566 people, mostly black, until the end of that year. Such revolutionary actions during this period were further bolstered by the ANC's 1985 Kabwe congress in Zambia that called on its supporters to make South Africa ungovernable.

The ages of these cohorts range between 35 and 60 and their years of birth range from 1948 to 1973. Interestingly but controversially, some social commentators also refer to this generation as *the lost generation* (see Seekings, 1996, also for a critique).

Post-Apartheid South Africa generations

The third period, representing grand- and great grandchildren with ages ranging from 13 to 26, covers the post-Apartheid period. These participants were born between 1982 and 1995 and the majority of these participants – Mandela's children[3] – spent most of their formative years in a liberated democratic South Africa, commencing with the presidency of Nelson Mandela.

★　★　★

The findings of the research reported in this chapter are strongly indicative of the recognition of the collective ideal of reciprocal support by both the older as well as the younger generations. The respective generations, however, depart from different perspectives towards this ideal. Older carers (mainly women) contribute support despite the circumstances – they are motivated by the notion that younger generations should always enjoy precedence. Contrary to this notion, the younger generations argue that support to older generations is to be mediated by the context: competing priorities on their time and resources will determine whether they render support to older generations. These differential obligations and priorities often leave older carers particularly vulnerable in terms of their own future care outcomes. Younger generations, moreover, increasingly perceive institutional care as a viable care option. The moral space between the perceived normative ideal and the pragmatics of the moment provides the scope for negotiation to regenerate or to contest the care relationship and is the focus of this chapter.

South African context

In the (South) African context, the relevance of family, intergenerational relationships and support/care is particularly defined by three current interrelated trends: population ageing, poverty-related government policies on the extension of social assistance and HIV/AIDS.

Population ageing

On mainland SSA, South Africa is the country with the highest proportion of older people and may overall be described as in the intermediate stage of population ageing (Kinsella and Phillips, 2005). With a total population of around 52 million, 4.1 million (8.2 per cent) is aged 60 and over. This older population is projected to increase to 5.23 million (10.5 per cent) by 2025 and by 2050 to 6.4 million, which will represent 13 per cent of the total population. The age group 80 years and older represents 9 per cent of the older population in 2011 and is projected to increase to 19 per cent by the middle of the century (Statistics South Africa, 2012; Actuarial Society of South Africa (ASSA), 2011).

The diverse nature of ageing patterns in the multi-ethnic society of South Africa with its multitude of social contexts is however masked by such a general description. It is therefore important to note that rates of population ageing across the three main demographic drivers – fertility, mortality and migration – vary among the respective racial groups of South Africa. Under Apartheid, the population was classified into four racial categories, namely black Africans, Whites, Coloureds[4] and Indians/Asians, with Whites particularly advantaged. This remnant from Apartheid – since dismantled with the 1994-democratic elections – still influences any understanding and analysis of the South African population, which is currently constituted by about 79.5 per cent black Africans, 9 per cent Whites, 9 per cent Coloureds, and 2.5 per cent Indians/Asians (Statistics South Africa, 2014). Of the 60 and older population, Whites constitute 26 per cent, Coloureds 5 per cent, and Indians/Asians 4 per cent. Despite the fact that black African older people constitute only 4.8 per cent of the total population, they do represent 64 per cent of the older cohorts and this chapter will focus on this particular group. The absolute number of black African older persons is furthermore expected to increase in coming decades, which will, because of their continued socio-economic disadvantage, have significant implications for future care management and service provision (Statistics South Africa, 2012).

The major tendency is that around 72 per cent of the non-institutionalised older population,[5] across racial groups, live in multigenerational households where they co-reside with children and/or grandchildren. By far the majority of these multigenerational households are headed by female black African older people, which make them particularly pivotal in intergenerational support (Statistics South Africa, 2012).

With its proportionately high number of working-age people and proportionately low number of young and old, South Africa should be in a position to take advantage of a demographic dividend (South Africa (Republic), 2011). However, entrenched poverty/unemployment and HIV/AIDS have resulted in many more dependants than would normally have been the case, highlighting the challenge of both upward and downward intergenerational support and care, including a lack of capacity.

Poverty and social protection in South Africa

The 2015 *Human Development Report* of the UN Human Development Index ranks South Africa 116th out of 188 positions having considered life expectancy, adult literacy, school enrolment rates and income (UNDP, 2015). South Africa is a middle-income country with one of the highest levels of economic inequality in the world. Poverty and entrenched inequality – on racial and gender grounds – are legacies of previous policies related to colonialism and Apartheid (South Africa (Republic), 2013; Bhorat et al, 2001).

Unemployment in South Africa is furthermore widespread, currently remaining around 36 per cent based on the expanded definition of unemployment, which takes discouraged work-seekers into account. It is youth unemployment (below the age of 35) that is particularly perturbing: respectively affecting 29.5 per cent (15–24-year olds) and 42.8 per cent (25–34-year olds) in 2012. For specifically black African youth, the unemployment rate is a staggering 65 per cent (South Africa (Republic), 2013).

Poverty, exacerbated by HIV/AIDS, and constitutionally guaranteed access to social security set the scene for the South African government to currently oversee, along with Brazil, one of the most rapidly expanding social welfare systems in the developing world – characterised by its near-universal coverage and relative generosity (Lund, 2008; Barrientos et al, 2003; Ferreira, 1999). The first 5 years of the new millennium saw the number of social grant beneficiaries in South Africa increased from just below 3 million to nearly 11 million. Currently, around 16.3 million of a population of some 52 million receive a social grant (South Africa (Republic), 2013). These state cash transfers provide a safety net for the poorest and serve a redistributive function to rectify economic and social inequities inflicted on the poor in the past (Lund, 2008).

The four social assistance programmes in post-Apartheid South Africa that provide the largest benefits and have the widest spread are the Old Age Pension (OAP), the Disability Grant, the Foster Care Grant and the Child Support Grant[6] (see Lund, 2008 for an in-depth discussion). As beneficiaries in one of only seven countries in SSA[7] to provide social pensions, the majority of older South Africans receive a non-contributory pension. This is a means-tested grant paid to some 2.7 million women and men from the age of 60,[8] worth approximately £80 per month. Although paid to individuals, benefits are pooled and redistributed – especially by black African females – at household and community levels (Ferreira, 2006a; 2004a; 2004b; Barrientos et al, 2003; Sagner and Mtati, 1999). In a 2002-study of the role of the OAP in alleviating poverty in the Eastern and Western Cape, 86.7 per cent of households indicated that they share resources and generally provide childcare and care for disabled, ill and unemployed individuals or members in the household. Over 81.3 per cent pensioners indicated that they retained none of the pension money for their own use, while a further 18 per cent said that only a 'little' or 'some' of the money was for their own use (Møller and Ferreira, 2003).

From the implementation of the OAP (1928), African pensioners were under considerable moral and normative pressure to share their pensions with kin and kith. A decision not to share the pension money would be interpreted as morally provocative and almost a denial of kin relationships. As Sagner and Mtati (1999) suggest: pension-sharing slots into this moral notion of kinship. It is intimately tied to a cultural ethos that emphasises the value of interdependence and the priority of family welfare over self-interest.

In spite of the strengths and the evolving nature of the social grant system in South Africa, the focus is only on those who are 'supposed' to be economically inactive, namely children, older people and those with disabilities. There is an obvious gap in the safety net for unemployed persons between 18 and 60 years. Given South Africa's high unemployment rate and the fact that only 3 per cent of the unemployed have access to unemployment benefits at any given time, the majority of school leavers from poor households will be unemployed and dependent on the transfers of those who are beneficiaries of a grant (South Africa (Republic), 2013). Considering the impact of HIV/AIDS, these 'goodwill transfers' also extend to care in the broader sense of the word where particularly older generations manage the care of their ill children and/or affected grandchildren.

HIV/AIDS

South Africa is one of the hardest-hit countries, with around 6 million people living with HIV/AIDS (UNAIDS, 2010; Lopez et al, 2006; Kinsella and Phillips, 2005). The distinctive feature of HIV/AIDS is the concentrated toll it takes on young adults in the prime of their productive and reproductive lives. This toll tends to cluster within the intimate space of families (with partners infecting each other and the virus also being transmitted to new-borns) and the long-term generational momentum that such epidemics can develop affect both ascending and descending generations.

USAID's analysis of DHS and MICS data (2004, 20) indicates that a high proportion of orphans live in households headed by older people (mostly grandmothers) – up to 60 per cent (also see Makiwane et al, 2004; UNICEF, 2003). Older people are indeed increasingly affected – and also infected – by HIV/AIDS. More recently, an increasing number of older people have been found to be infected with HIV; many more, infected earlier, may be expected to develop AIDS as successive age cohorts enter the older age groups (see Ferreira, 2006b). Older people do not enter routine (for example ante-natal) surveillance systems (confined to women aged 15–49 years), and thus have limited opportunities for detection, diagnosis, treatment and counselling. They are also excluded from global estimates of the disease, which further obfuscates their risk of infection (Joint United Nations Programme on HIV/AIDS and World Health Organization (UNAIDS/WHO), 2007; HelpAge International, 2005; Albone and Cain, 2008). With virtually no institutional care options for AIDS patients or orphans, and in most cases not even considered, poor grandmother-headed networks in particular have ultimately to provide the necessary shelter and care in-house (see Ferreira, 2006b for an overview).

The contemporary core Emalahleni care narrative

Against this backdrop of entrenched poverty and massive unemployment in South Africa, the care for both HIV/AIDS-infected and -affected younger generations dictates a focus on the asymmetrical downward support by older generations for younger generations. In turn, however, the realities of downward support relate to the expectations of future upward support of older generations. More specifically, this part of the chapter will reconstruct a core narrative of the realities of current intergenerational relationships and its implications for future care of older people as perceived by Emalahleni older generations within the contemporary moment and affirmed or contested by younger generations in the relevant multi-generational networks. This reconstruction of a core narrative does not seek to provide evidence of a generalised pattern; it remains a story with many variations within and across these multi-generational networks. These individual first level narratives, grounded in people's lived experiences, however, lead a core Emalahleni story beyond microfication. Based on current intergenerational patterns, the Emalahleni account on present and future care implies neither uniformity in participants' experiences, nor a predictable general sequential pattern, but conceptually offers three broad cross-cutting and intertwined storylines, namely the normative ideal, the relational pragmatics of the contemporary moment and the moral space (lag) in-between.

The normative ideal (the told story)

Superficially and at first impression it would seem that older (G1/G2) and younger generations (G2/G3/G4) position themselves at opposite sides of the continuum in relation to tradition. The Emalahleni narrative, however, strongly indicates that both older and younger generations recognise and affirm the collective ideal of familial solidarity and reciprocal support. This explains the response Winnie [79 – G1] received from her family in trying to deal with her difficult grandchild [Lerato, 25 – G3]:

> Winnie [G1]: The family can also see that things are not right, but… if we say that Lerato should leave, they just say: 'No, our father and the ancestors will be unhappy

with that.' They say that it's her own life, I have to accept that. When she's gone, maybe only for two weeks, they will blame me. It's very difficult. They say I must stay with her – that is our culture. It's a sin [to forsake somebody] because no matter what she does to one, don't forsake her. It is not about me; it is about her.

Similarly the comment of Charles [17 – G4] about his great-grandmother [83 – G1]:

Charles [G4]: Our tradition says that one should not leave one's children – the ancestors will haunt you. If, for example, you are employed you will be losing your job. Things will fall down for you. But on the opposite side, like my grandmother, God will extend her days. The ancestors will welcome her with an open hand. The ancestors want us to be reunited with our children so that their ways will be brighter.

My granny is very good to us. She does so many things – she buys us stationery, clothes and much more. She thinks before I can even ask. I am very happy living here, her cleaning of the house, the food. Even if she is not able to cope anymore, she will still continue. I also do some cleaning. I feel obliged to do something back.

They depart from the ideal where the rhythmic drum-beat of generalised reciprocity lies at the core of intergenerational relationships. Both these older and younger generations explicitly and implicitly agree that, where needed and for as long as needed, older generations must support younger generations. Likewise they agree that ideally older generations should be supported by younger generations to reciprocate the care and support they received and currently enjoy from such older generations (if so). The general value of assisting older relatives (or relatives in general) and the obligation to support older parents clearly persist and are endorsed by the young. Point of the told (albeit performed) story is: an overall endorsement of the normative ideal of solidarity across different response patterns and different generations. Clear indications of shifting or weakening mutual intergenerational support norms and attitudes are less evident. All generations display (perform) resilience on the normative level: 'Yes, that is the way it should be.'

Relational pragmatics: impacting and mediating factors (the lived story)

All the respective interviewed Emalahleni generations have a collective normative bottom line: a broad adherence to filial obligation norms and the ideal towards intergenerational solidarity. However, in implementing the ideal, the generations depart from different positions depending on their disordered life cycles. Whereas the Emalahleni older generations see their support as more prescriptive, a duty-bound, even sacrificial obligation, whatever the context may be, the younger generations see their reciprocal support more in terms of a flexible range of guidelines with limitations, depending on the circumstances when and as fitting (see Freeman, Chapter Five).

It is found that older carers contribute support *despite* the impact of circumstances ('I must, even if I don't want to') – their motivation being that younger generations should always enjoy precedence over the oldest generation (also see Van Eeuwijk, Chapter Three, footnotes 8 and 11). The following Emalahleni quotes illustrate the Zulu saying: *Abantwana babantwana bami bafana nezingane zami* (These are my grandchildren, these are my child's children, so whatever life brings with it, I have to take it).

> *Sarah* [G1]: They do not respect me. They waste the food and I am tired of them. I wish they will just go away...But who am I going to give them [the grandchildren] to? I have to struggle. Nobody will look after them! It is because they are mine!

> *Martie* [G1]: Where are they [grandchildren] going to live? Because they don't work; they don't have anything – no food. What are they going to do?...I have to live here to take care of them and take control of them. If there is something to be done I have to tell them and... [yap like a little dog]...
> But if I will eat nice and sleep OK, it's not going to work. I must keep everybody going.
> I just have to do it. As I light two candles and pray to God, I often ask what I have done to suffer like this: the rent is too high and there is no food. But...if I think clearly, I think of the children's father and then I know I can't throw away his children. I often ask God to help me so that I can live here until I die. Then if they know that

their mother died then they can suffer on their own; they will make plans to live.

These older carers argue from the stance of 'I must' in spite of limited resources and capacity – demonstrating a duty that overrides capacity and context. Although future expected reciprocity plays a role, these older carers' motivation seems to go far beyond generalised reciprocity. Especially since their contributions seem to acquire a character of sacrifice that might not necessarily (even knowingly) be reciprocated. In general, older generations (especially women) experience high degrees of pressure and tend to pursue a discourse of sacrifice and victimisation where the younger generations (especially teenage and mature grandchildren) are perceived to be the perpetrators.

In practical terms, the contributing carer is *mutatis mutandis* the sacrificing carer. Something along the lines of what Land and Rose (1985) understand as the 'compulsory altruism' of care – the tension between the duty of self-sacrifice for the sake of the younger dependant and the rights/needs of the carer, leaving them insecure about their own future care as something not to be taken for granted.

For their part, younger generations argue that support to older generations is *mediated by* circumstances: care/support is limited to the extent that they are in a position to, and as it corresponds with the hierarchy of their current and future priorities ['I can't, even if I want to'] as illustrated by Busi's comments.

> *Busi* [G2]: That is how it should be: first the parent should take care of the children, but when the parent gets old someone who's working and has money, whether it is the eldest or not they should take the responsibility. We as children must care because it is our mother. She always looked after us. Tradition says children have to care, but it doesn't work like that – the one that has work – that one [child/grandchild] will have to do it. But we have to care… it also depends on the personality.

Younger generations argue from the departure point of capacity and hierarchy of needs. This holds that in situations in which resources are constrained, the needs of immediate family (children, spouse and older parents) have clear priority over those of more extended kin; and, what is more important, the needs of the young (self, spouse and children) have priority over those of older parents. If and when older people do in fact receive some measure of material support from younger generations, the initiatives are generally infrequent and small. Although not specifically mentioned by the second generation, the idea of care by way of placing an older person in an old-age home and at the same time pursuing a career is a recurring theme in the third generation. In their eyes this does not necessarily imply an abandonment of the normative obligation of care for older generations, but a pragmatic approach to reconfigure and balance care responsibilities with possible future career opportunities necessary for survival of all. This is illustrated by Thabisile's [24] comments about future care of older members in her multi-generational household.

> *Thabisile* [G4]: Yes, I think that's no problem to one day care for my grandmother.

She, however, immediately qualifies her response once her grandmother left the room.

> But I don't think that other young people think in the same way, because there is a lot of work to do once you decide to care for somebody. It depends on the individual. Sometimes, like when my grandmother is not here, I must care for my great-grandmother and then I must wake up in the middle of the night for her and my friends would say 'No, never!' People's circumstances change and I think there is nothing wrong to take granny to the old-age home, because say we get a job and maybe we all go to work in the morning...We can't leave old people by themselves, so there is a place for an old-age home. Sometimes they are not happy because they want to live with their grandchildren but there they bathe them and give them food. They take good care of them. If I get a job, I will try and explain it to my mother or my grandmother. Then I will take her there.

Moral space of negotiation: towards regeneration of the ideal

In the space generated between the collective ideal and the pragmatics of the moment, relationships are negotiated, reconfigured, regenerated and/or contested. So, in general the Emalahleni older carers (irrespective of gender) negotiate in terms of a cyclical downward pacifying of younger generations within the network while younger generations are more orientated towards a linier dialectic of rights and progress (see Stroeken, 2008).

Although older carers cannot conceive their lives without these younger generations, they would have preferred to have been able to lead a less complicated and more autonomous existence. This is, however, not the reality in a resource-constrained context. Thus, the Emalahleni older generations have instead developed a complaint discourse to keep the younger generations (and others) informed about the ideal they envisage as illustrated by Antjie [78].

Antjie [G2]: One day, they will care for me because they see what I do. I will, however, not be able to say exactly who I think will eventually do it. They [she points to the younger ones] must not know otherwise they will not pull their weight now [they laugh]. In my heart I know, but that thing will remain in my heart.

I try to be an example for my children and their children; they must learn from that. Yes, they must look after me for the grandchildren to see. Lately they take old people to the old-age home. My mother's sister went there. But I don't want to. Lots of people said the house will not be clean when there are older people, so I must wash her and bathe her. But [laughs] I think they don't love their mother. If you love your mother, you will not chase her away. And other young people don't like older people; they don't want them because they don't like them.

At the same time, older carers in these situations can only but anticipate and negotiate their own care as illustrated by Martie [84].

Martie [G1]: It is the last-born that is supposed to care. He gets the house and he should care. Sydney is the last-born, but actually I know that it will be Tryfina [living in Klarinet, nearby]. She is my child number three. I was ill once and she did everything. So I saw that this child loves me with her heart ... The children at Middelburg don't help. They cannot; they have children of their own; maybe bring something small if they come to visit.

The position of the generations in relation to one another is determined by their position in the life course and their capacity in the negotiation process. Although their pensioner status put some older generations at an asymmetrical advantage in terms of financial capacity in relation to younger generations, they are at an asymmetrical disadvantage given the conditionality and the limitations built into the generational contract. These limitations on the normative level imply that younger generations are obliged to provide filial support *only* if they are in a position to do so. As soon as support of aged parents/relatives starts to infringe on adult children's responsibilities to their immediate family (self, spouses and children) or available capacity, a normative hierarchy of priorities and family obligations come into effect. These limitations are further strengthened by an assumption that older generations have no right to use the resources that the young need, even if this is detrimental to their own welfare in favour of the young (for a historical overview see Sagner, 2001 and Moffat, 1842, 136).

From a normative as well as a pragmatic point of view, the contemporary Emalahleni care contracts intrinsically position older generations as vulnerable in relation to younger generations, particularly in resource-constrained situations (see Pype, Chapter Two, p 43). In all these patterns the entrapped vulnerability of older carers and the frustration of younger generations are evident. It can consequently be hypothesised that continuous downward support of younger generations by older generations in resource-constrained contexts is a precursor for entrenched vulnerability regarding their own future care – more so if it is exacerbated by HIV/AIDS.

Against this background and given the differential positions of the respective generations and the conditions and limitations determining the nature of these relationships, older participants are nevertheless highly creative and pragmatic in interpreting, negotiating and responding to the ideal of intergenerational solidarity.

> *Min* [G1]: People are not controlled by tradition any more, especially the children. You should sit down, look at your situation and then decide.

It is essentially this notion of relativity and conditionality – with older generations thinking or suspecting that their downward support will for various reasons not necessarily be reciprocated – that drives them to negotiate from a more autonomous–pragmatic position. Within the basic mode of survival, the architecture of these responses within all the Emalahleni multi-generational families presents itself dynamically in two distinct but intertwined matrices: an internal one which draws on kin and kith and an external one that draws on, when available, diverse external options. These matrices, in any conceivable configuration, revolve around ideas and practices of *cash* and *care* whereby cash generally refers to material support and care to the more instrumental/socio-emotional support.

Two complementing patterns of dedicated tailor-made internal and external care patterns negotiated by all older participants emerge in some or other (re)configuration, namely by: either openly identifying a chosen younger individual to take responsibility for current and future care needs and expectations, or complementing the internal matrix with available external support matrices.

Openly identifying a chosen younger individual to take responsibility for current and future care needs and expectations

To have some notion of future security/stability (control) within a highly flexible context, most of these older participants project their care expectations on a particular younger individual – the chosen one – to support them in their current situation and/or potentially take care of them in the future (thus attempting to regenerate the normative ideal).

> *Angel* [G1]: It's because of the way she [May – her daughter] took care of me and also cares for her sisters and brothers. When we can go traditionally they would have said it's [care] a must but when we force someone to do it, it is not going to work. It must come from the heart. Tradition is only a force. You must rather look at the way a child is behaving. You see, this generation is not the same as the generation before them. But some still do that – only some specific families.

Martie [84] similarly illustrates this when she considers her future: '*I know their hearts.*' She then refers specifically to her daughter: '*Her heart is warm. Her heart is in the right place. I look at their faces and then I see their hearts.*' Referring to her son, however, she is realistic too: '*I don't want to say too much but I see his heart. I see that I bother [irritate] him.*'

A few older participants even invest in or indulge very small children, with a specific aim to win them or their parents over. Their deliberate strategy is to create an emotional and material dependency. In certain contexts it is as if the older person wants to start a new cycle of reciprocity all over again. Min [51] illustrates the process of strategically initiating such a new reciprocal care cycle. Her 'investments' in her foster child is based purely on reciprocal consideration for the future;

not on blood or tradition, but on gratitude (also see Freeman, Chapter Five).

> *Min* [G1]: I know that tradition says you should be cared for by your own blood but I think if it is not your own blood it is best. Because when you tell her [Busi, a 2-year old orphan] that you saved her and cared for her, she will be thankful and one day care for you. She will not take things for granted because she is not your own blood. Things lately depend more on the particular family than the tradition. People are not controlled by tradition any more, especially the children. You should sit down, look at your situation and then decide. Families are not the same. Each family must deal with their own situation. It is the way they are acting, the way I see them.

The rationale behind her thinking is disappointment with all her children's earlier behaviour, taking her for granted and not respecting her. Her perception is that they are less inclined to contribute to the common good of the immediate network.

The selection and choice of a particular individual can indeed be immensely complex and in some cases the older people furtively identify a younger individual and keep the whole multi-generational network in anticipation.

Complementing the internal matrix with available external support matrices

All the older participants complement their internal care/support arrangements with additional external arrangements. Older participants thus generate supplementary kin–kith relations and relationships of support to fulfil their unique needs, as many lost one or more children through accidents, *the disease* (HIV/AIDS) or other causes and/or have no hope of any capacity within existing networks. In order to broaden their range of support options to regenerate the collective ideal, they have all established additional external networks with various degrees of success. Different configurations of these internal/external care matrices are possible, with some participants involved in literally all the available external networks in that community, namely the church, the Mthimkhulu Centre and Housing for the Aged, government programmes and facilities and an array of relief charities and friends (also see Pype, Chapter Two and Van Eeuwijk, Chapter Three). Apart from the programmes and facilities provided for older people by the government, including the OAP and an array of health services, these external networks are utilised to provide support on all levels, but especially emotional support as expressed by Martie [84]:

> If I am at home, I think about the children too much; my heart doesn't get any rest. There, at the church and when I am at Mthimkhulu, my head and my heart open up.

Older carers themselves negotiate and construct pragmatic internal and complementing external matrices to keep the collective ideal alive. They live this ideal by selecting, within the internal matrix, the appropriate individual according to their needs and/or by constructing complementary alternative communities within their peer group network. Because families and kin are often seen as not providing adequate care, they seek alternative locations for care, such as churches where they generate an alternative ethos around the collective ideal (see Klaits, 2001).

Conclusion

Much of the research on issues of care focus on questions of stress and the burden of downward support, leaving older carers vulnerable in terms of their own care needs – especially those older carers in the fourth phase of the life course. All these tensions have not, as suggested by Durham and Klaits (2002), necessarily resulted in making kinship irrelevant but are instead altering the strength of certain relationships.

Little attention is paid to questions of care for older people, however. There has been no systematic documentation of how care for older people is provided, nor is there active discussion on what the relative care roles and responsibilities of families, the state and other sectors should be. There is little systematic documentation of care needs of older people, the amount and type of care received or the impact on older people and their families of unmet care needs. A key reason for the lack of enquiry and debate is an overriding official discourse, which declares the centrality of the family in the care for older people as an unassailable African value and model as well as the NGO-driven contribution discourse (AU/HAI, 2003; African Union, 2004; African Union, 2006; HAI, 2011).

The findings of this research provide glimpses of two competing processes at work with regard to current and future care for vulnerable older people:

Scenario 1

Here, older people would prefer to relinquish (albeit reluctantly) co-residence within the multi-generational household to be accommodated in some form of institutional care. This is resisted by younger generations on the basis of the performed discourse about the care of older people within the family circle. However, in actual fact and more mundanely, the discourse often masks a fear of losing the regular OAP income. Most institutional care in South Africa needs a percentage of the OAP to subsidise it, causing the intergenerational network to lose out on much-needed income.

Scenario 2

Younger generations (especially G3) increasingly explore the idea of some form of formal care for older people, not necessarily approved by the older generation. The pragmatic argument of the younger generations is that they essentially still care, but need these facilities/services for the care of older people to be able to pursue employment opportunities – of great importance in a resource-constrained and survivalist context. If capacity is in any event so depleted as a result of poverty and HIV/AIDS, formal, even institutional care is seen as a viable option. This resonates with Croll's (2008, 109) review of ethnographic studies on ageing in Asia, which depicts younger generations' reinterpretation of filial support as modified to relate more to 'support, service and care based on need, volunteerism and mutual appreciation, gratitude and affection', instead of 'piety, obedience or duty'.

This, given younger generations' dependence on the monthly pension income of the older person, clearly has major implications for the dependent younger generations. On the one hand, younger generations see external care options and support networks to which they can entrust the care of the oldest members in need as a pragmatic solution to fulfil their own care obligations. At the same time this gives them the freedom to pursue their own quest for autonomy and to pursue the limited employment opportunities available. On the other hand, while unemployed the younger generations remain dependent on the older person's (especially women) current or future pension and they need to physically keep these older pensioners (contributors) within the multi-generational household for as long as possible. If employed these young people would, however, prefer the older person to spend their days either at the service centre or be admitted to an old-age home, especially if the older person is in need of specialised care. In general these external care possibilities put dependent younger generations in an ambivalent position: between complementary care support and the loss of material resources in the form of the OAP.

New interpretations and modifications of the meanings and practice of filial piety are being developed, showing influence of local circumstances of history, economics, social organisation and demography, and personal circumstances of wealth, gender and family configurations (Ikels, 2004, 2).

Multi-generational livelihoods imply a differential positioning with regard to the relationships of which the respective generations are part – not only given their respective different developmental stages in the life course (including the impact of HIV/AIDS) but also concerning the way in which each generation respectively experiences and understands their being (their meaning-making) in the world at the particular time of this study.

Ideally, over the life course, the early sacrifices of motherhood should later be rewarded with meaningful care in old age, but this dynamic is increasingly under strain and uncertain. Socioeconomic and epidemiological pressures, furthermore, pose extreme challenges to intergenerational relationships and the ways in which they are already being reconfigured. Emalahleni's older generations find themselves in an intrinsically vulnerable position regarding their own future care needs.

Notes

[1] The terms 'care' and 'support' will be used interchangeably in this chapter.

[2] An analysis where the perceptions of the respective generations are explored at the interface of both its familial and historical meanings. In this way an in-depth view is achieved within and across generations through an analysis of the current intergenerational dynamics.

[3] 'Mandela's children', as used here, does not refer to the specific longitudinal study *Mandela's children: Growing up in post-Apartheid South Africa* that followed the lives of Soweto children born in the year of his release (Barbarin and Richter, 2001).

[4] The term 'Coloured' was used to represent a specific ethnic group in South Africa whose origins date back more than 350 years and refers to an ethnic group of complex mixed origins. The term is retained by South Africa's Statistical Office within its formal classification system of the country's four main racial groups.

⁵ Although South Africa is the only country in SSA with a developed formal care system for older persons, due to Apartheid few residential care facilities were available to black African older persons in the past – however, since the end of Apartheid, such facilities are accessible to all. There are an estimated 44,000 subsidised beds available for frail older persons.

⁶ Other grants include the Care Dependency Grant, which assists parents of a disabled child (0–18 years) who requires care at home by another person. When such a child reaches the age of 18, application must be made for the adult Disability Grant. The Grant-in-Aid is an additional grant awarded to persons who are in receipt of the OAP, Disability, or War Veteran's Grants, and who are unable to care for themselves.

⁷ Other countries are Botswana, Lesotho, Swaziland, Mauritius, Namibia and most recently, Zanzibar.

⁸ The age-eligibility criterion for men was lowered to 60 years as from 1 April 2008.

References

African Union, 2004, *Plan of Action on the Family*, 16 July, http://sa.au. int/en/sites/default/files/plan_of_action_on_the_family-16july2004. pdf

African Union, 2006, *African Youth Charter*, 2 July, http:///www.unhcr. org/refworld/docid/493fe0b72.html

AU/HAI (African Union/HelpAge International), 2003, *The African Policy framework and plan of action on ageing*, Nairobi, Kenya: HelpAge International Africa Regional Development Centre

Albone, R, Cain, E, 2008, *Mind the gap: HIV and AIDS and older people in Africa*, London: HelpAge International

ASSA (Actuarial Society of South Africa), 2011, *Demographic scenarios*, Unpublished report for the National Planning Commission (NPC), Pretoria: NPC

Barbarin, O, Richter, L, 2001, *Mandela's children: Growing up in post-Apartheid South Africa*, New York: Routledge

Barrientos, A, Ferreira, M, Gorman, M, Heslop, A, Legido-Quigley, H, Lloyd-Sherlock, P, Møller, V, Saboia, J, Werneck, MLT, 2003, *Non-contributory pensions and poverty prevention: A comparative study of South Africa and Brazil*, London: HelpAge International and Institute for Development Policy and Management

Bhorat, H, Leibbrandt, M, Maziya, M, Van der Berg, S, Woolard, I, 2001, *Fighting poverty: Labour markets and inequality in South Africa*, Landsdowne, South Africa: UCT Press

Croll, E, 2008, The intergenerational contract in the changing Asian family, in R Goodman, S Harper (eds) *Ageing in Asia*, pp 473–91, London: Routledge

Durham, D, Klaits, F, 2002, Funerals and the public space of sentiment in Botswana, *Journal of Southern African Studies*, 28, 777–95

Ferreira, M, 1999, The generosity and universality of South Africa's social pension system, *The EU Courier* 176, 55–6

Ferreira, M, 2004a, Born in the Eastern Cape and now a social pensioner, in M Ferreira, E Van Dongen (eds) *Untold stories: Giving voice to the lives of older persons in new South African society. An anthology*, pp 25–41, Cape Town: University of Cape Town, Institute of Ageing in Africa

Ferreira, M, 2004b, The social old age pension: A fundamental gift of economic and social power to older persons, *Les Cahiers de la FIAPA* 3, 158–66

Ferreira, M, 2006a, The differential impact of social-pension income on household poverty alleviation in three South African ethnic groups, *Ageing and Society* 26, 337–54

Ferreira, M, 2006b, HIV/AIDS and older people in sub-Saharan Africa: Towards a policy framework, *Global ageing: Issues and action* 4, 2, 56–71

HAI (HelpAge International), 2005, *The frontline: Supporting older carers of people living with HIV/AIDS and orphaned children in Mozambique, South Africa and Sudan*, London: HAI

HAI (HelpAge International), 2011, *Ageing in Africa* 36, 1–12, London: HAI, http:///www.helpage.org/resources/publications

Ikels, C (ed), 2004, *Filial piety: Practice and discourse in contemporary East Asia*, Palo Alto, CA: Stanford University Press

Kahn, RL, Antonucci, TC, 1980, Convoys over the life course: Attachment, roles, and social support, in PB Baltes, O Brim (eds) *Life-span development and behavior*, Vol 3, pp 253–68, New York: Academic Press

Kinsella, K, Phillips, D, 2005, Global aging: The challenge of success, *Population Bulletin* 60, 1, 40

Klaits, F, 2001, *Housing the spirit, hearing the voice: Care and kinship in an apostolic church during Botswana's time of AIDS*, Unpublished PhD thesis, Boston, MA: Johns Hopkins University

Land, H, Rose, H, 1985, Compulsory altruism for some or an altruistic society for all?, in P Bean, J Ferris, D Whynes (eds.) *In defence of welfare*, pp 74–96, London: Tavistock

Lopez, AD, Begg, S, Bos, E, 2006, Demographic and epidemiological characteristics of major regions, 1990–2001, in AD Lopez, CD Mathers, M Ezzati et al (eds) *Global burden of disease and risk factors*, pp 15–44, New York: Oxford University Press

Lund, F, 2008, *Changing social policy: The child support grant in South Africa*, Cape Town: HSRC Press

Makiwane, M, Schneider, M, Gopane, M, 2004, *Experiences and needs of older persons in Mpumalanga*, Pretoria: Human Sciences Research Council

Moffat, R, 1842, *Missionary labours and scenes in Southern Africa*, London: J Snow

Møller, V, Ferreira, M, 2003, *Getting by…benefits of non-contributory pension income for older South African households*, Cape Town: University of Cape Town, Institute of Ageing in Africa

Ramphele, M, 1993, *A bed called home: Life in the migrant labour hostels of Cape Town*, Cape Town and Johannesburg: David Philips

Sagner, A, 2001, 'The abandoned mother': Ageing, old age and missionaries in early and mid-nineteenth-century South-East Africa, *Journal of African History* 42, 173–98

Sagner, A, Mtati, RZ, 1999, Politics of pension sharing in urban South Africa, *Ageing and Society* 19, 4, 393–416

Seekings, J, 1996, The 'lost generation': South Africa's 'youth problem' in the early 1990s, *Transformation,* 29: 103–25

South Africa (Republic), 2011, *National development plan: Vision for 2030*, Pretoria: National Planning Commission, The Presidency

South Africa (Republic), 2012, *White Paper on Families in South Africa*, Draft, Pretoria: Department of Social Development, www.dsd.gov.za/index2.php?option=com_docman&task

South Africa (Republic), 2013, *Budget Review, 2013*, Pretoria: National Treasury

Statistics South Africa, 2012, *Census 2011: Highlights of key results*, www.statssa.gov.za/census/census_2011/census_products/Census_2011_Methodology_and_Highlights_of_key_results.pdf

Stroeken, K, 2008, Tanzania's new generation: The power and tragedy of a concept, in E Alber, S Van der Geest, SR Whyte (eds) *Generations in Africa: Connections and conflict*, pp 289–308, New Brunswick, NJ and London: Transcation Publishers

UNAIDS, 2010, *UNAIDS report on the global AIDS epidemic 2010*, New York: UNAIDS

UNAIDS/WHO (Joint United Nations Programme on HIV/AIDS and World Health Organization), 2007, *AIDS epidemic update*, New York: UN

UNICEF, 2003, *Africa's orphaned generations*, New York: UNICEF
UNDP (United Nations Development Programme), 2012, *Report on the millennium development goals (MDGs)*, New York: UNDP
UNDP (United Nations Development Programme), 2015, *Human development report. Work for Human Development*, New York: UNDP
UNPD (United Nations Population Division), 2011, *World population prospects: The 2010 revision*, New York: UNPD, www.un.org/en/development/desa/publications/world-population-prospects-the-2010-revision.html
USAID (United States Agency for International Development), 2004, *Sub-national distribution and situation of orphans: An analysis of the president's emergency plan for AIDS relief focus countries*, Washington, DC: USAID

Afterword:
Discourses of care for older people in Sub-Saharan Africa: towards conceptual development

Andries Baart

> In Mr Coetzee's story, the mother tells her son to be careful with language. '*Take care of*...Be careful, John. In some circles take care of means *dispose of*, means *put down*, means *give a humane death*.' (Douglas, 2013, emphasis in original)

This collection presents fascinating, alarming, yet appealing research. Even a superficial reading of the chapters in this volume suggests enormous dilemmas in providing social and health care for older people in contemporary Sub-Saharan Africa (SSA) – now, at this moment, and even more so in the near future. Whose priority is care provision? Where should funding come from? What is needed in terms of good care? (What is good care anyway?) Where can necessary capacities be found? Who is helping and who should be? What of older people's responsibilities to take care of themselves? Who is ultimately responsible or should be made accountable? What are actual care practices? All these questions are essential to our understanding of care in SSA, but after a deep reading of all the respective contributions the overarching question is: what is the meaning of all of this on a broader more conceptual level? How do we bridge the gap between this mostly descriptive, localised research and a common discourse on good but affordable long-term care for older people in need? As raised in the Introduction, how do we transcend the increasing tendency of microfication of social research on ageing as pointed out by Hagestad and Dannefer (2001)?

In order to develop at least a starting point towards a common discourse of contemporary care *for* older people in SSA, my immediate aim is to offer, based on the contributions in this volume as a unit of analysis, a conceptual next step by utilising discourse analyses to better understand the challenges of long-term care for older people in SSA towards possible interventions. I draw on the French philosopher Michel Foucault (1977; 1980; 2003) who, step by step, developed a concept of discourse that can be summarised as: 'systems of thoughts composed of ideas, attitudes, courses of action, beliefs and practices that systematically construct the subjects and the worlds of which they speak' (see Lessa, 2006). The Foucaultian version of discourse (Foucault, 1970; 1972) presupposes the inextricable knotting of language use, the expression of meaning, the exercise of power, the claim of knowledge, and the constitution of practices. It is essential Foucault to trace the role of discourse in wider social processes of legitimisation and power. In so doing Foucault then focuses on the *construction of current truths* – how they are maintained and what power relations they carry with them. Discourses occur and mutually overlap in a complex way within practices (Bourdieu, 1977; 1991; Nicolini, 2012; Schmidt, 2012; Schatzki, 1996; Reckwitz, 2002; Bueger and Gadinger 2014). Foucault (1977; 1980; 2003) repeatedly stated that power is always present and is able to both produce and constrain the truth. Discourses exert power by operating, essentially, through rules of exclusion. Given the focus of this volume, it is also important to note that there is a direct link between discourse and space. According to modern German phenomenologists (Schmitz, 2007) the relation of subject and space may be described as taking your place in a space, and the movement within your space. This concept of discourse will be the lens with which the narratives in this volume will be analysed. Its focus thus chiefly concerns:

- *critical discourse analysis* (CDA) rather than specific linguistic varieties of discourse research, including a strictly linguistic analysis of speech and conversation;
- *discourse analysis* (DA) as a *means to an end* rather than as an end in itself (Cameron, 2001, 7); *interdisciplinary* rather than mono-disciplinary types of DA;
- (within the domain of the CDA) *epistemology* rather than power structures *per se*; the dominance of ideas rather than the controlling influence of political power;
- *written* language ('grey literature') rather than spoken language.

Discourses on care in this volume

To generate a common discourse on care for older people in need, the main questions are: what themes and patterns can be discerned, and which narrative lines give them coherence?

By (re)constructing *discursive formations* in the texts and their sources, as well as taking into account the practices that produce and are produced by these discourses, the relevant themes have been listed, patterns within those themes were looked at, after which those patterns were listed into clusters until all data were covered. This resulted in six types of surface 'stories', or six visible lines of reasoning, which act as 'discursive formations'. These six discursive formations are followed by a discussion of four discourses that underpin these surface stories.

To assign meaning to each of these discursive formations, I designated a term for each based on one of their central variables: the motive for providing care (for older people). In this way I have identified six core discursive formations, which are designated as follows:

- conventional habits;
- personal engagement;
- formal opportunity;
- trained solidarity;
- market mechanism;
- improvisational effort to 'save' one-self.

These above-mentioned discursive formations are now explained in greater detail, preceded by a summarised table (Table A.1) containing the themes explored. Subsequently, their mutual relations are determined, and lastly the underlying discourses are identified.

Discursive formations

For the sake of clarification it is important to include two preliminary notes:

- As mentioned above, I selected *relevant themes* to identify the discourses. Although all the chapters in this volume have presented rich data, not every detail has been included. The decision about which data to include proved a contentious one. Because of the particular focus of this volume, that is, care *for* older people in SSA, criteria for selection were themes that contained possible indications about the nature of the care provided. Some of the stories elaborated on the personal histories of the care receivers, but general biographical and more personal information about individual care receivers were not included in the analysis. Individual complaints and needs issues are not altogether less relevant; this is why I included information on the kind of care older people *expected* to receive, as

Table A.1: The six discursive formations in this volume

Caring because of...→ ↓ Variables	1. Conventional habits	2. Personal engagement	3. Formal opportunity	4. Trained solidarity	5. Market mechanism	6. Improvisational effort to save one self
1. Varieties	From effective to contested	From moral virtues to personal image improvement	From service by state to service by NGOs	From community complement to professional supplement	From free to regulated market	From individual self-management to cooperation of mutual interest
2. Origin	Culturally anchored conventions and practices	Lived or felt moral obligation, whether or not with intention of personal profit	Formal, bureaucratic institutional arrangements	Educational programmes	Formal contract of mutual profit	Collapse of resources
3. Perspective on caring	Historical: obedience to social positions	Intentional: appropriated motivation of individual carer	Provision: availability of professional carers	Community: availability of voluntary carers	Systemic logic of exchange of contract parties	Vulnerable elderly without help
4. Form	(No longer) taken for granted in specific traditions	Ethical sensitivity and conviction, whether or not mixed with well-understood self-interest	General services for who meets the formal terms of being included in the service	To be trained as responsible member of the community and as the 'prolonged' arm of the professional regime	Trade: money for service	Muddling through
5. Level of aggregation	Collective ('the African way of caring')	Personal or individual and on voluntary basis	Impersonal but collective	Partial/some specific cohorts or non-motivated or non-participating residents	Exchanging parties per service type	Individual or little, opportune 'cooperation'

Caring because of... → ↓ Variables	1. Conventional habits	2. Personal engagement	3. Formal opportunity	4. Trained solidarity	5. Market mechanism	6. Improvisational effort to save one self
6. Prerequisite	Plausible and favourable tradition	Moral sensitive, compassionate people, whether or not with calculated self-interest	Capable, well-funded institutions with bureaucratic mediated access	Room, programmes, and tools for training volunteers or caring family members	Well-functioning market system	Capable and not too frail elderly
7. Who does it?	By tradition or convention appointed parties: those in the objective position to care	Everybody with high moral standards and good reasons to practice them	Paid professional carers	NGOs and other community 'workers': they empower and activate others to care	Supplying and demanding parties, whether or not in conjunction with the social community	Help yourself!
8. Solidarity	Mechanical solidarity	Affective/selective solidarity	Abstract/general solidarity	Instructed, local solidarity	Solidarity of interests	Cooperative solidarity
9. Strengthened by	Traditional thinking and cultivating traditional philosophy	Moral authorities (churches, religion, authoritative opinion leaders)	Policy of government or NGOs	Community building programmes promoting practical solidarity and mutuality	Systemic coordination of care	Empowerment policy
10. Direction	Care comes in due course to care entitled persons	Care searches needy persons	Indigent searches care	Care takes shape in the interaction of willing carers and empowered care receivers	Care is result of negotiation	Care is self-provided
11. Kind of care	Caring about and caring that	Caring that and caring about	Caring that	Caring that and caring about	Caring that	Caring that

Caring because of.... → ↓Variables	1. Conventional habits	2. Personal engagement	3. Formal opportunity	4. Trained solidarity	5. Market mechanism	6. Improvisational effort to save one self
12. Broadness of care	All kinds of care, help, support, incl. honour/respect	Care within the ethical universe of provider's preferences	Programme-oriented and bureaucratic mediated care delivery	Additional care (lacking in the community or professional regime)	Only affordable care	Emphasis on basic care for survival
13. Danger	Ideological rhetoric: huge gap between adhered to ideal and empirical reality	Instrumental abuse of moral motives; decreasing role moral authorities; patronising and too much based on self-interest	Weak institutions, deficient opportunities and low or no care priority for older persons: westernisation: care sees residential models of first and second world	Bad connection/ no suitable effective educational curricula	Creaming: only for the well-off; meritocratic logic	Acceptance injustice, dishonourable position of needy ones
14. Who receives care?	Respected persons	Chosen persons	Needy persons	Fellow citizens	Who pays for it	Self-reliant persons
15. Space as place of care	Traditional community and family	Value community	Welfare state: dispersed facilities	Reconstructed community of fellow residents	Market (personalised at home)	Social margins and social exclusion: unprotected public sphere
Phenomenological formulated	Elderly in centre, time is (hi)story	Motives at the surface, time to act	Facilities in foreground, time to go to the background	Communal life at the surface, time to live together	Contracts in the centre; time is money	Elderly in background, margin and below horizon; survival time

Caring because of... → ↓ Variables	1. Conventional habits	2. Personal engagement	3. Formal opportunity	4. Trained solidarity	5. Market mechanism	6. Improvisational effort to save one self
16. Space as domain of care	Cultural space, connected to identity and honour	Symbolic space, connected to preciousness of human life	Provisional space, connected to civil rights and justice	Social space, connected to living well together	Economic space, connected to freedom of (rational) choice	Physical space, connected to endurance and survival
17. Space as room for care	Decreasing/against evidence and (high/spate) modernity	Decreasing but with potentials; modern motives for altruism?	Small but increasing see western welfare models	Increasable but in need of realistic and rigorous modernization of curricula	Increasing but vulnerable: (too) capitalistic model?	Increasing by fate: desperate measure
18. Manipulable by social interventions?	– – Shrinking and losing acceptability: hard to steer, influence, or slow down	+/– Transforming and renewing itself, may be fostered and facilitated because of its idealistic potentials	+ Upcoming, seems inevitable, modern development, but looked at with suspicion and mistrust	++ Stimulated and well programmable: in rhythm/pace, direction and acceptability could best connect to life world and its discursivity	– Repulsing home-grown solutions, quite demanding for young states but powerful: self-regulating	+/– Symbolise the powerlessness of existing care institutions but may be transformed by empowering programmes

well as regarding their efforts and trajectories for obtaining it (or not). However, my focus was on the more general discourses, keeping in mind that historical information is mostly relevant (Foucault's 'genealogy') but the local colouring less so.

• The discursive formations were ordered by motive, as care, more often than not, is underpinned by different configurations of motives. Some of these motives link up effortlessly; others are contradictory and contest one another. At this point it is essential to understand that identifying distinctive motives does not imply that people only have one motive for caring, or that the identified 'discursive formations' could be valued 'on their own'.

Table A.1 should be read both vertically and horizontally. An overall view (vertical reading) of Table A.1, rows 1–14 could be interpreted as follows:

1 Conventional habits

The narrative here underpins the kind of care[1] that is provided on the basis of taken-for-granted conventions and (moral and religious) habits, that is, on the basis of tradition, traditional positions, responsibilities, dependency relations and the willingness of people to do what they are expected to do. Here we have the so-called 'African way of caring' – an enclosed practice. When 'tradition' is contested (as is increasingly the case, as reflected in this volume) the provision of care is pressurised and goes hand-in-hand with impossible demands, frustration and neglect, to the point where no care at all might be provided (see Chapters One, Two and Six). In the classical sense the presumed solidarity is 'mechanical' (see Émile Durkheim). This care should be seen as all-encompassing and includes honouring older people; it consists of 'caring that' (the essential things are done) and 'caring about' (giving emotional support, being attentive, and so on).[2] One need not ask for this care nor search for it, ideally it should come to you in due time *if you have earned it* (as an older person you may lose your entitlement if you don't behave according to convention). The story of this kind of care can easily become rhetorical; it readily transforms into ideology, an effort to make believe, and can happen for any number of reasons: policy, self-interest, performativity, shame, adherence to traditions, or the desire for power (see Chapters One, Three and Seven).

2 Personal engagement

The second discursive formation is around personal engagement: an individual's acknowledged motivation for caring. It overlaps with 'conventional habits' and contains two storylines (see Chapters Two and Seven): (a) the moral (virtuous) altruistic motive, and (b) the well-understood motive of self-interest, that is to say donors who wish to improve their image by making public donations. Caring or not-caring is predominantly a personal decision, whether it is in line or in conflict with tradition. The solidarity involved is selective: one chooses whom to care for and whom to reject. Personal affections and preferences are undeniably involved in the practices of this discursive formation. Similarly, the content of care is a personal choice: what does not fit into the moral universe or intentions of the carer is not provided. Moral authorities may influence the development of a certain amount of sensitivity and willingness, but this 'receptiveness to influence' may be abused too: in such case personal motives are instrumentally used for extrinsic purposes. The ambiguous, unstable and highly personal character of the motive to care/to donate could be seen as potentially patronising, but it may also be a testimony of either incredible dedication or radical disinterestedness. This type of care looks actively for people who are in need of it and its basic direction is towards 'the other'. It is not a case where the person who needs care should find it for him- or herself, anywhere, and anyhow.

3 Formal opportunity

The third discursive formation relates to providing accessible care services on a broad basis, either by the state or by NGOs. Some of these services are already operationalised, or will be realised shortly; they are mutually competitive or in a complementary relationship. Although there may be important overlaps, care here is largely disconnected from traditional thinking, as well as from personal motives and intentions. Care provision is operationalised and practised by formal organisations with bureaucratic procedures ('Are you indigent enough?') and by professionals. It is rather impersonal, but intended to be fair, and mostly based on rights and supposedly accountable procedures. The emphasis is not necessarily on 'caring that' but on 'caring about'. Normally, in such cases, the needy person has to find his own way to the care and through a jungle of conditions, procedures, and so on. Solidarity here has an abstract and anonymous character: by paying taxes, supporting faith-based organisations financially, and donating to charitable organisations, one may demonstrate solidarity. Such care may seriously suffer from bureaucracy, lack of means, weak programmes and management, or even be seen as patronising and based on the 'westernisation of care institutions'.

4 Trained solidarity

'Trained solidarity' appears to be a relatively weak narrative in this volume, but not in terms of the background literature nor as a practice. Care provision is stimulated by large-scale (re)educational programmes for local communities and general advocacy initiatives with the aim of finding and training family members, neighbours, fellow residents, and volunteers to care for each other, including caring for lonely, needy, older people (see Chapter Three). Essential in this case are the community workers and the educational programmes that should motivate and generate organisational structures, as well as enough capacity to offer 'home-grown' programmes and actual care delivery. To develop such practical solidarity a successful appeal must be lodged in terms of citizenship, being a fellow man, or being collectively responsible for good life in the local community. This kind of care may overlap with more formal services and even with personal engagements and traditional caring patterns, which is quite possible given the right flexibility and organisation. To this end, the underlying ideas ('discursivity') of leading a good life together need to be critically cultivated and further developed. What kinds of care are to be provided and how should this be determined through the mutual interactions of the people involved? The latter produce particular practices and their lives, conversely, are produced by these practices. This type of care provision fails when good and effective educational programmes are lacking, but also when service delivery is usurped by professionals and the 'volunteer community', who disappoint in its provision, are missing in action, or think they have other issues to pursue.

5 Market mechanism

Another, understandingly, rather weak narrative in this volume is that of the neo-liberal market (Biebricher 2012) that regulates care provision (see Chapters One and Two). This market may be totally free (capitalistic), or may be stringently regulated by the state, in which case it may be effectively linked to the discursive formations of 'formal opportunities' and even to 'trained solidarity'. In contrast with the previous discursive formations, the central purpose is not care but, essentially, profit. The relationship here is not based on compassion but on contractual agreements, while the distribution mechanism is that of demand and supply. What kind of care will be delivered rests heavily on what is needed, paid for and deliverable. The coordination is non-personal and systemic; it is to be negotiated. Here, care is for those who can afford it, with solidarity grounded in common interest. A major disadvantage may be the tendency 'to cream', that is to only care about the well-to-do with no investment in complex, risky or even incorrigible needy people. In the market's idiom, caring for these needy people with all the complexities accompanying them often results in what could be seen as failure; wasted energy and loss of honour (the needy cause the carers to fail and to look like losers).

6 Improvisational effort to save oneself

In this volume there are also stories of older people without any decent care: where traditional care provision totally fails (children lacking means, opportunity, motivation, endurance, and so on); where there are no accessible formal care services in proximity, no financial means to buy what is needed; where people might wander from shelter to former husband, to the next nephew, to an open field, and so on (see Chapters One to Seven). They lack facilities; they are not welcome; they cannot be tolerated (due to their complaints, 'madness', demanding behaviours, or illness). And if they choose to live (or end up) in a residents' home, they suffer from prejudice and mythical imaginaries. Such homes are the perceived places of witches and the devil. Nevertheless, within this gloomy narrative (practice) is another story told from the perspective of vulnerable elderly people without help: being self-reliant, muddling through, being streetwise, 'helping yourself', creating togetherness ('cooperations'), and being gifted with the inventive art of improvisation and resilience. The emphasis is on survival and being strong enough (or at least 'physically empowered') to take care of oneself. If one succeeds, one has to deal with the next menace, namely society's acceptance of such deplorable, dishonourable, care.

This concludes a general reading of Table A.1, rows 1–14. In rows 15–17 the question of space (one of this volume's objectives) is addressed. Row 18 offers suggestions about the future by addressing the question of whether or not these practices and discursive formations are open to social interventions and 'improvements'.

Convergence, coherence and conflict

As already mentioned, these six discursive formations naturally overlap and partially presuppose one another – Figure A.1 sketches out their relations.

Figure A.1: The relations of the discursive formations

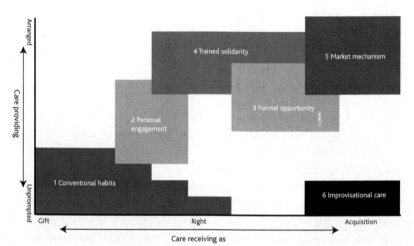

On the *horizontal* axis the variable is how frail older people get the care they need. On one end care is a gift, and on the other something one has to acquire with one's own efforts (begging for it, meeting bureaucratic criteria, paying for it). Between these two extremes, care could be seen as a right – partially a gift and partially an attainment. On the *vertical* axis the variable is how care is provided, and ranges from fairly spontaneous modes to conscious arrangements. Unsolicited care is provided on a taken-for-granted basis in terms of who should provide it, what the care should be like, when ought it to be offered, and who is entitled to it. Arranged care depends on reflectiveness, (moral) deliberation, and is located within the framework of existing policies (or their lack); it also depends on training and the building of appropriate structures. Therefore, the quadrangle in which the respective discursive formations are placed is restricted by the possible values of 'care receiving' and 'care providing'. Each of these positions will now be looked at in detail.

Conventional habits (1) could be placed low on the left side. This does not imply that such 'habits' are practised without arrangements, but they slope down towards the middle (towards rights). From this position three lines of care receiving/providing can be identified:

- developments in which discursiveness plays an important role as a means to arrange care (*top centre*);
- developments that are much more systemic and where abstract, rather impersonal, coordinating mechanisms are used to negotiate care (*right upper corner*);
- developments that result from neglect, which are neither discursively nor systemically regulated (*right corner at the bottom*).

The other discursive formations are also now placed in the quadrangle along these three lines. Personal engagement (2) and trained solidarity (4) are in line with the more communicative developments, both deeply rooted in traditional, moral thinking. Personal engagement (2) and trained solidarity (4) also interrelate, and personal engagement (2), furthermore, overlaps with both conventional habits (1) and trained solidarity (4), which in a way connects them both. Although it has many characteristics of the spontaneous gift, it represents, on one hand, a halfway ('artificial') arrangement, and on the other, a ('natural') spontaneity, as it gradually moves in the direction of 'rights'. Trained solidarity (4) – a totally arranged mode of caring – is the link between the communicative and systemic lines of development, straddling both domains. It overlaps with personal engagement (2) and on the other hand (actually rather heavily) with formal opportunity (3) and market mechanism (5). The training programmes presuppose a certain degree of personal motivation and intents, in order to result in some accessible and fair caring structures. The line of systemic developments is mainly 'occupied' by formal opportunity (3) and market mechanism (5), both with substantial overlaps. Both are also characterised by 'acquisition', as is 'improvisational care' (6), be it because of neglect or its totally offhand nature.

Discourses

These discursive formations and their mutual interrelatedness can now be analysed from the perspective of our focus, namely discourses. What is the meaning behind the language? What are the 'hidden' statements and what kind of (power) practices are exposed?

In this analysis the following four discourses are discussed in more detail (Figure A.2).

A. The *cultural-conformable discourse* is generally underpinned by two discursive formations, namely 'conventional habits' and 'personal engagement'. This discourse is essentially conservative and requires

Figure A.2: Four discourses in this volume

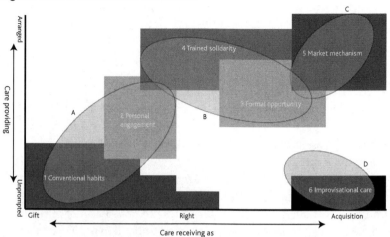

matters to be kept as they have always been: the positions of older people, the significance of honour, the habit of doing the expected good to older people, and so on. The orientation of this discourse is the past and its main resource is moral-cultural capital (see Chapter Seven). The exercise of power takes the shape of omnipresent pressure, expectations and complaints repeatedly uttered in order to conform to a so-called traditional behaviour. In this discourse the interaction with reality is on the level of ideology: what ought to prevail. Tradition is the most important source of social position, rights and obligations; and agency ensues from the extended family.

B. The *structural-adaptive discourse* includes the third and fourth discursive formations ('formal opportunity' and 'trained solidarity') but also touches upon 'personal engagement' and 'market mechanism'. Its orientation is pragmatic and developmental: the creation of fit for purpose structures for caring in the near future. Its main 'currency' is social capital and competence. Power takes the form of persuasion and elicitation to participate in development through discursiveness and interventions. Although ideas and ideals are encompassed within it, its interaction with the complex reality is empirical and implies the competent implementation of what works and has satisfactory effects. The agency rests with the community, whether local social entities or more universal/general formations like the state or NGOs. Care is distributed, not on the basis of traditional positions, but on the basis of rights and needs.

C. The *calculating-innovative discourse* is transformative in that it breaks with the traditional, communitarian and moral orientations of care provision. It overlaps greatly with the discursive formation of 'market mechanisms' but also has a clear intersection with the structural-adaptive discourse. It is aimed at the future and therefore builds primarily on financial capital and skilled expertise. Power is exerted in the constant pressure to adjust to neoliberal systemic requirements, represented as the inevitability of late modernity. This discourse has a complex relationship with reality but its essence relates to the commodification of care – care is business and has quality standards equal to those of for-profit institutions. The actor (care receiver) is the autonomous individual, who is in a position to make rational choices, and who gets what he deserves. In this context neither complaints nor a nostalgic looking back to the past will be rewarded, but being strong, competitive and self-reliant will.

D. The *functional-subsistence discourse* concurs with the 'improvisational care' discursive formation but is probably wider, as future research still has to explore. It is the discourse on ousting and withdrawal related to older people's active or passive non-participation in care-receiving. Their orientation is not to the future or the past, but toward survival in the actual here and now. They have just one resource or asset at their disposal: physical capital in close relation with streetwise inventiveness. Power here is predominantly located in the capacity to resist and refuse, and in being deviant. In this discourse interaction with reality mainly takes the form of retreating and vetoing in order to avoid repetitive pain and distress. The actor is – as in the preceding discourse – 'autonomous', but in this case in the mode of being isolated and self-reliant. What he gets is what he arranges for himself.

The four discourses portrayed here are deeply connected with different practices of caring, and are internalised in (a lack of) institutions, policies and social identities. They nevertheless occur simultaneously, and are intertwined within the same contexts. They (mostly implicitly) battle one another for domination. These above-identified discourses may offer a basis for exploring care options.

Although there are no convenient and confident quick fixes, the preceding analysis offers potential for teasing out some ideas about the challenges of caring for older people in SSA. Drawing on this preceding discourse analysis, the approach of discursive institutionalism, as developed by Schmidt (2008; 2013), seems to offer possibilities for a way out and, in conclusion, needs to be explored for future reference.

In 2008 Schmidt wrote a substantial article in which she systematically summarises and elaborates this idea of discursive institutionalism in a nutshell (p 302):

> The turn to ideas and discourse in political science has come to constitute a fourth 'new institutionalism'. I call it discursive institutionalism (DI), distinct from rational choice institutionalism (RI), historical institutionalism (HI), and sociological institutionalism (SI). Political scientists whose work fits the DI rubric tend to have four things in common. First, they take ideas and discourse seriously, even though their definitions of ideas and uses of discourse vary widely. Second, they set ideas and discourse in institutional context, following along the lines of one or another of the three older new institutionalisms, which serve as background information. Third, they put ideas into their 'meaning context' while they see discourse as following a 'logic of communication,' despite differences in what may be communicated how and where. Finally, and most importantly, they take a more dynamic view of change, in which ideas and discourse overcome obstacles that the three more equilibrium-focused and static older institutionalisms posit as insurmountable. What most clearly differentiates discursive institutionalists from one another is not their basic approach to ideas and discourse but rather the kinds of questions they ask and the problems they seek to resolve, which tend to come from the institutionalist tradition(s) with which they engage.

In 2013, in *Does discourse matter in the politics of building social pacts on social protection?* Schmidt adds:

> The discursive interactions may involve policy actors in discourse coalitions, epistemic communities, and advocacy coalitions engaged in a 'coordinative' discourse of policy construction as well as political actors engaged in a 'communicative' discourse of deliberation, contestation, and legitimisation of the policies with the public. Such 'communicative action' may involve informed publics of the media, opinion leaders, intellectuals, experts, and 'policy forums' of organized interests as well as the more general public of ordinary people and civil society.

In researching social policy development in SSA, Kpessa and Béland (2013) warn insistently against copying and pasting European or western models in analysing social problems, change and government. They nevertheless conclude their article with an explicit approval of explanatory theories, including discursive ('ideational') institutionalism (italics are mine, AB):

> the core causal factors identified by industrialisation scholars, power resource theorists, historical institutionalists, and *ideational and cultural researchers* should remain central to any attempt to provide a systematic explanation of social policy trends in SSA countries…[C]ausal factors associated with the four theories need to be re-evaluated and interpreted with SSA's unique historical experiences in mind. (p 336)

This contribution, which began with discourse, also ends with it: discourses matter, and should be understood and taken seriously as bases for a solid understanding and interpretation of politics and political change. I conclude with a comment by Berman (2001, 247) in a review article in the hope that this afterword, based on the preceding chapters will at least offer a prompt for the serious study of care for older people in SSA:

> In a period of rapid political change, when the old rules can no longer be taken for granted, some political scientists have returned to the study of ideational variables. However, for the contemporary ideational renaissance to fulfil its promise and continue to help scholars better understand political life, its adherents need to accept greater systematisation and theoretical rigour.

Notes

[1] I use the term '*conventional* habits' for this discursive formation in order to distinguish it from psychological or behavioural habits. 'Traditional habits' is a less adequate formulation: within tradition there are more specific (local) conventions.

[2] There are many varieties in the literature, but this difference is essential: 'caring that…' is oriented towards things to do, to tasks. In expressions like 'caring for', and even more 'caring of' and 'caring about' the care is oriented to people who need care: (a) the needy person is important and relevant for me, (b) I take responsibility for caring

in a practical sense, and (c) I feel or develop an inner emotional and moral commitment to do so. That difference between 'task-orientated' and 'person-orientated' care is, whatever the precise formulation, the point I wish to make.

References

Berman, S, 2001, Ideas, norms, and culture in political analysis, Review Article, *Comparative Politics* 33, 2, 231–50

Biebricher, T, 2012, *Neoliberalismus, zur Einführung*, Hamburg: Junius Verlag

Bourdieu, P, 1977, *Outline of a theory of practice*, New York: Cambridge University Press

Bourdieu, P, 1991, *Language and symbolic power*, Cambridge, MA: Harvard University Press

Bueger, C, Gadinger, F, 2014, *International practice theory: New perspectives*, Houndmills: Palgrave Macmillan

Cameron, D, 2001, *Working with spoken discourse*, London: SAGE

Douglas, S, 2013, The Nobel-winning novelist and the sculptor: How Berlinde De Bruyckere got JM Coetzee to curate the Belgian pavilion. 'Cripplewood' gets at the darker side of Venice, *Observer/ Culture*, 5 May

Foucault, M, 1970, *The order of things*, New York: Pantheon

Foucault, M, 1972, *Archaeology of knowledge*, New York: Pantheon

Foucault, M, 1977, *Discipline and punish*, New York: Pantheon

Foucault, M, 1980, Two lectures, in C Gordon (ed) *Power/Knowledge: Selected interviews*, New York: Pantheon

Foucault, M, 2003, *Society must be defended*, New York: Picador

Hagestad, GO, Dannefer, D, 2001, Concepts and theories of aging: Beyond micro-fication in social sciences approaches, in RH Binstock, L George (eds), *Handbook of aging and social sciences*, San Diego, CA: Academic

Kpessa, MW, Béland, D, 2013, Mapping social policy development in sub-Saharan Africa, *Policy Studies* 34, 3, 326–41

Lessa, I, 2006, Discursive struggles within social welfare: Restaging teen motherhood. *British Journal of Social Work* 36, 2, 283-98

Nicolini, D, 2012, *Practice theory, work and organization*, Oxford: Oxford University Press

Reckwitz, A, 2002, Toward a theory of social practices: A development in culturalist theorizing, *European Journal of Social Theory* 5, 243–63

Schatzki, TR, 1996, *Social practices: A Wittgensteinian approach to human activity and the social*, Cambridge: Cambridge University Press

Schmidt, R, 2012, *Soziologie der Praktiken: Konzeptionelle Studien und Empirische Analysen*, Berlin: Suhrkamp

Schmidt, VA, 1996, *From state to market? The transformation of French business and government*, New York and London: Cambridge University Press

Schmidt, VA, 2000, Values and discourse in the politics of adjustment, in FW Scharpf, VA Schmidt (eds) *Welfare and work in the open economy, Vol I: From vulnerability to competitiveness*, pp 229–309, Oxford: Oxford University Press

Schmidt, VA, 2002, *The futures of European capitalism*, Oxford: Oxford University Press

Schmidt, VA, 2003, How, where, and when does discourse matter in small states' welfare state adjustment?, *New Political Economy* 8, 1, 127–46

Schmidt, VA, 2006, *Democracy in Europe: The EU and national polities*, Oxford: Oxford University Press

Schmidt, VA, 2008, Discursive institutionalism: The explanatory power of ideas and discourse, *Annual Review of Political Science* 11, 303–26

Schmidt, VA, 2009, Putting the political back into political economy by bringing the state back yet again, *World Politics* 61, 3, 516–48

Schmidt, VA, 2010a, Taking ideas *and* discourse seriously: Explaining change through discursive institutionalism as the fourth new institutionalism, *European Political Science Review* 2, 1, 1–25

Schmidt, VA, 2010b, On putting ideas into perspective: Schmidt on Kessler, Martin and Hudson, and Smith, in A Gofas, C Hay (eds) *The role of ideas in political analysis: A portrait of contemporary debates*, pp 187–203, London: Routledge

Schmidt, VA, 2013, *Does discourse matter in the politics of building social pacts on social protection? International experiences*, Santiago: ECLAC United Nations, *Series Social Policy* #178, http://repositorio.cepal.org/bitstream/handle/11362/6194/S2013800_en.pdf

Schmitz, H, 2007, *Der Leib, der Raum und die Gefühle*. Bielefeld/Locarno: Aisthenis Verlag

Van Dijk, TA, 1995, Discourse analysis as ideology analysis, in C Schäffner, A Wenden (eds) *Language and peace*, pp 17–33, Aldershot: Dartmouth Publishing

Waldenfels, B, 2009, *Ortsverschiebungen, Zeitverschiebungen. Modi leibhaftiger Erfahrung*, Frankfurt: Suhrkamp Verlag

Index